# RETHINKING SEXUAL AND REPRODUCTIVE HEALTH AND RIGHTS FOR YOUNG WOMEN IN SOUTHERN AFRICA

This important book provides a critical examination of the sexual and reproductive health and rights (SRHR) of young women and girls in Southern Africa, examining the ways in which current policies and programmes aimed at improving SRHR often fail to reach the most marginalised populations.

Addressing key regional challenges such as high rates of HIV, unintended pregnancies, unsafe abortions, and sexual and gender-based violence, the book highlights how health inequalities in the region are in fact increasing, despite the 2030 Agenda for Sustainable Development of "leaving no one behind". The book draws on theoretical analysis and empirical data gathered from studies carried out in five Southern African countries (Madagascar, Mozambique, South Africa, Zambia, and Zimbabwe), arguing that a continued focus on HIV and interventions that target health in a narrow sense often fail to understand the wider socio-economic determinants of poor sexual and reproductive health and the ways in which girls and young women are made vulnerable.

Written by leading scholars in the field, this will be essential reading for students and researchers in Global Health, International Development, Women's Studies, and all related fields.

**Tamaryn L. Crankshaw** is a senior research fellow and leads the SRHR Programme at the Health Economics and HIV and AIDS Research Division (HEARD) at the University of KwaZulu-Natal, South Africa.

**Jane Freedman** is a Professor at the Université of Paris 8, France, and Director of the Paris Centre for Sociological and Political Research (CRESPPA).

**Carolien Aantjes** is a senior research fellow at HEARD at the University of KwaZulu-Natal, South Africa, and a senior researcher in the Access to Justice research group of the Inholland University of Applied Sciences in Rotterdam, the Netherlands.

**Nana K. Poku** is the Vice-Chancellor and Principal of the University of KwaZulu-Natal (UKZN), South Africa, and Executive Director at the Health Economics and HIV and AIDS Research Division (HEARD) at UKZN.

## Routledge Global Health Series

Series Editors: Nana K. Poku and Jane Freedman

This timely series provides robust and multi-disciplinary assessments of the actors and dynamics shaping the health of humanity under globalized and still globalizing conditions. Books in the series come from a range of disciplinary perspectives in order to address the complex interactions of human and natural systems and the roles of governments and international organisations in protecting the health of their citizens.

The series welcomes full proposals, outlines and general queries on all themes and issues pertinent to global health. This includes medical, political, sociological, and economic perspectives on health, health governance and health finance; poverty and insecurity; the prevention and treatment of important but under-researched diseases; gender and health; the implications of global pandemics; and the varieties and challenges posed by the growing, worldwide expectation of some form/degree of Universal Health Coverage.

**Migrant Health and Resilience**
Transnational Competence in Conflict and Climate Displacement Situations
*Peter H. Koehn, Phyllis Bo-yuen Ngai, Juha I. Uitto, Diana M. Diaków and Susan Martin*

**Rethinking Sexual and Reproductive Health and Rights for Young Women in Southern Africa**
A Critical Perspective
*Tamaryn L. Crankshaw, Jane Freedman, Carolien Aantjes and Nana K. Poku*

For more information about this series, please visit: https://www.routledge.com/Routledge-Global-Health-Series/book-series/RGHES?srsltid=AfmBOooSW8iiRALbkBdklYbRz6ePA7NKT47w5aHcoNeuNIGWxEWul2Wp

# RETHINKING SEXUAL AND REPRODUCTIVE HEALTH AND RIGHTS FOR YOUNG WOMEN IN SOUTHERN AFRICA

## A Critical Perspective

*Tamaryn L. Crankshaw, Jane Freedman, Carolien Aantjes, and Nana K. Poku*

Routledge
Taylor & Francis Group
LONDON AND NEW YORK

Designed cover image: Getty Images

First published 2025
by Routledge
4 Park Square, Milton Park, Abingdon, Oxon OX14 4RN

and by Routledge
605 Third Avenue, New York, NY 10158

*Routledge is an imprint of the Taylor & Francis Group, an informa business*



*British Library Cataloguing-in-Publication Data*
A catalogue record for this book is available from the British Library

*Library of Congress Cataloging-in-Publication Data*
Names: Crankshaw, Tamaryn, author. | Freedman, Jane, author. | Aantjes, Carolien, author. | Poku, Nana, 1971- author.
Title: Rethinking sexual and reproductive health and rights for young women in Southern Africa : a critical perspective / Tamaryn Crankshaw, Jane Freedman, Carolien Aantjes and Nana K Poku.
Description: Abingdon, Oxon ; New York, NY : Routledge, 2025. | Includes bibliographical references and index.
Identifiers: LCCN 2024025937 (print) | LCCN 2024025938 (ebook) | ISBN 9781032540108 (hardback) | ISBN 9781032540078 (paperback) | ISBN 9781003414698 (ebook)
Subjects: LCSH: Reproductive rights--Africa, Southern. | Women's rights--Africa, Southern. | Women's health services--Africa, Southern.
Classification: LCC HQ1236.5.A356 C73 2025 (print) | LCC HQ1236.5.A356 (ebook) | DDC 362.1/98100968--dc23/eng/20240628
LC record available at https://lccn.loc.gov/2024025937
LC ebook record available at https://lccn.loc.gov/2024025938

ISBN: 978-1-032-54010-8 (hbk)
ISBN: 978-1-032-54007-8 (pbk)
ISBN: 978-1-003-41469-8 (ebk)

DOI: 10.4324/9781003414698

Typeset in Times New Roman
by KnowledgeWorks Global Ltd.

# CONTENTS

# ABOUT THE AUTHORS

**Tamaryn L. Crankshaw** is a senior research fellow and leads the SRHR Programme at the Health Economics and HIV and AIDS Research Division (HEARD) at the University of KwaZulu-Natal, South Africa.

**Jane Freedman** is a Professor at the Université of Paris 8, France, and Director of the Paris Centre for Sociological and Political Research (CRESPPA).

**Carolien Aantjes** is a senior research fellow at HEARD at the University of KwaZulu-Natal, South Africa, and a senior researcher in the Access to Justice research group of the Inholland University of Applied Sciences in Rotterdam, the Netherlands.

**Nana K. Poku** is the Vice-Chancellor and Principal of the University of KwaZulu-Natal (UKZN), South Africa, and Executive Director at the Health Economics and HIV and AIDS Research Division (HEARD) at UKZN.

# ACKNOWLEDGEMENTS

We would like to thank all our colleagues with whom we have worked over the past years and without whom we would not have been able to write this book. Special thanks go to Victoria M. Mutambara, Mina Rakotoarindrasata, Jean de Dieu Randrianasolorivo, Yasmin Rajah, Samantha Chareka, Pemberai Zambezi, Nelson Muparamoto, Joseph Zulu, Mwali Banda, Ngamanya Nkunika, Tiki Banda, Khátia Munguambe, Vasco Muchanga, Rehana Capurchande, and Carlos Cuinhane.

We would also like to thank all of those who took time to respond to our questions and who took part in interviews and focus group discussions over the course of our various research projects. Without their precious inputs and insights, our work would not be possible.

The financial assistance of the Swedish International Development Agency (SIDA), the Ministry of Foreign Affairs of the Kingdom of The Netherlands (Grant number: 00091626) as part of their regional HIV/AIDS and SRHR programme in Southern Africa, and the South Africa/France PROTEA Programme (Grant Agreement number: 42390SL) is gratefully acknowledged. The content of the book, opinions expressed, and conclusions arrived at are solely the responsibility of the authors and do not necessarily represent the official views of the funding agencies.

# 1
# INTRODUCTION

## Introduction

The inspiration for this book arose from over a decade of research on the sexual and reproductive health and rights (SRHR) of adolescent girls and young women (AGYW) in Southern Africa, and many hours of discussion with young women in various countries in the region, as well as with colleagues from civil society organisations (CSOs) and with other researchers. Our various research projects working with AGYW of different social classes, ages, nationalities, and migration statuses in five Southern African countries pointed to the continuing impacts of gender inequality in their lives, which combines with other forms of inequality and discrimination to create situations of sometimes extreme vulnerability for them. We found, however, that existing frameworks for research (including our own) and policy often fail to appreciate the complex intersecting structures of inequality which lead to this vulnerability and are thus unable to identify those most marginalised and to propose adequate policies and interventions to ameliorate their situation and allow them to realise their rights and improve their health and well-being. This book was thus born of a certain frustration with these existing research and policy categories and frameworks, and a desire to go beyond them and to think more widely and more deeply about AGYW's SRHR in the region.

To give an example, one of the central research projects on which all the authors were engaged focused on young people who are considered "key populations" (groups who are supposedly more at risk of HIV infection) in five Southern African countries, looking at their SRHR vulnerabilities and policies to address these. We will discuss this project and the "key population" label

DOI: 10.4324/9781003414698-1

in more detail further in the book, but what we wish to highlight here are the limitations that we found in using this categorisation and the boundaries that these "key population" labels placed on our research. These limitations have pushed us to think and theorise more widely about vulnerability, how it can be defined and understood, and what this might mean for SRHR research and policy in the Southern African region, and more broadly. This research project started out using a group-based approach to vulnerability: identifying members of a pre-defined group such as sex workers, young people in detention etc. and assuming that being included in this group signified both a certain heterogeneity and similar experiences of vulnerability between group members. We began the research using this group-based approach to identifying vulnerability (the different ways of understanding vulnerability will be discussed further in Chapter 2) but quickly discovered that both differences within groups and similarities between those inside and outside these pre-defined categories severely limited our analysis and created artificial binaries that led to our project potentially overlooking those most vulnerable. Research with identified "sex workers", for example, led to potentially overlooking/neglecting the experiences of other young women involved in sexual-economic exchanges who could experience the same negative SRH outcomes but who did not identify as a sex worker and were thus not included in this group. Subsequent research projects with populations such as young refugee women pushed us further to question the ways in which social structures and systems of inequality create positions of vulnerability which are experienced differently by individuals located at different positions within these matrices of inequality. This pushed us to reflect further on how and why AGYW may be positioned in situations of vulnerability and how they might be supported to gain greater resilience. We will thus argue throughout the book that an approach focusing on "key populations" or "vulnerable groups" can result in a failure to identify and target those most marginalised in terms of their SRHR. In addition, the continuing focus on HIV from which the "key population" categorisation emerges may contribute to the sidelining of other pressing SRHR concerns faced by AGYW (such as sexual and gender-based violence) and to the overlooking of shared intersections of vulnerability (and opportunities for intervention), leading to not only poor HIV indicators but also other negative SRH outcomes.

SRHR have long been a major issue in global politics and have come to the forefront of debate following the closing of the era of the Millennium Development Goals (MDGs) and the United Nations General Assembly adopting a new development agenda in 2015 (United Nations General Assembly, 2015) that included a wide range of economic, social, and environmental objectives known as the Sustainable Development Goals (SDGs). Unlike the MDGs, the SDGs explicitly recognised SRH as being essential to health and development and women's empowerment. This led to the inclusion of two goals related to SRHR: SDG 3 (ensure healthy lives and promote well-being for all at all ages) and SDG 5 (achieve gender equality and empower all girls) and catalysed increased attention over how to ensure universal SRH care and to "leave no one behind". However, SRHR are also a highly contested set of issues, and despite the adoption by many policy-makers and researchers of the Guttmacher-Lancet Commission definition of SRHR in 2018 (Starrs et al., 2018), there is still a poor understanding of the scope of SRHR and how policies and interventions should be developed to improve health and rights. In this sense SRHR are open to different interpretations and SRHR policies may focus on a range of issues with varying weight accorded to each of these. In the case of sub-Saharan Africa (SSA), the scale and urgency of addressing the HIV pandemic has meant that responses to HIV have had a central structuring effect on the ways that SRH "risk" and vulnerability have been framed and understood. And frequently this has been done in a primarily "biomedical" way, which often reproduces colonialist and gendered framings of disease and infection and neglects wider structural and socially determined vulnerabilities.

We argue in this book that this framing and understanding may not always be sufficient to identify the most marginalised and vulnerable in terms of their SRHR or to deliver the most appropriate SRH services for them. As Sen et al. (2019, p. 321) argue, 'strategy frameworks on HIV/AIDS (sic) have advanced participation of people with AIDS, bringing attention to those most at risk of contracting HIV. However, there is failure to articulate an understanding of HIV as part of a broader SRHR agenda, while implementation has too often omitted marginalised groups'. Even after all this time and all the progress made, AGYW living in SSA continue to be disproportionately affected by a range of SRHR issues including HIV and early and unintended pregnancies, but also a whole range of other challenges and unmet needs which are not fully addressed by existing policies.

We aim to provide a more nuanced picture of the complex ways in which interacting social norms and political, legal, and economic structures create gendered inequalities in health and rights in different settings. Our empirical focus on Southern Africa will offer examples to illustrate the complex interactions of gender and SRHR on a continent where pressing preventable health issues persist, including high rates of early and unintended pregnancies, morbidity and mortality arising from unsafe abortion-related complications, HIV, and other sexually transmitted infections (STIs). Fundamental to this is the pervasiveness of sexual and gender-based violence (SGBV), which we address in Chapter 5. The region continues to contend with alarmingly high rates of SGBV, which directly and indirectly impacts women's (and their children's) health and well-being in profound ways. The difficulties in securing SRHR for all women, including the most marginalised, are not unique to Southern Africa, but in using our empirical research to analyse and illustrate the issues in this region, we hope to provide insights and recommendations both for the region and more globally.

## Sexual and Reproductive Health and Rights Are a Gendered Issue

'Why is it that something that is so fundamental to women ends up being the most controversial in the development agenda?' This question, asked by Helen Clarke, then Administrator of the United Nations Development Programme at a high-level meeting on SRHR in New York in 2014, is central in highlighting the fact that SRHR are unlike many other areas of health or social policy in the way that they have become points of contention and debate at international and national levels. Questions are raised not only about the practicalities of health service delivery or the best ways to improve SRH outcomes but also about the moral and ethical status of SRH choices and outcomes. Thus, these health services and rights, which are vital to well-being, are often difficult to access or even denied to many members of society, and this denial may be justified or legitimised by recourse to discourses that point to the illegality or immorality of certain behaviours and certain health procedures. What emerges is a system of what Morgan and Roberts label "reproductive governance", which 'refers to the mechanisms through which different historical configuration of actors – such as state, religious, and international financial institutions, non-governmental organisations (NGOs), and social movements – use legislative controls, economic inducements, moral injunctions, direct coercion, and ethical incitements to produce, monitor, and control reproductive behaviours and population practices' (Morgan & Roberts, 2012, p. 243). SRHR are clearly a gendered issue, impacting women to a far greater extent than men. As the Special Rapporteur on Health noted, 'There is no single cause of death and disability for men between the ages of fifteen and forty-four that is close to the magnitude of maternal death and disability' (United Nations General Assembly, 2006, p. 5). And yet women's health needs, particularly their SRHR needs, are still often denied or overlooked.

As Sen et al. (2020) argue, the realisation or non-realisation of SRHR is about power. Power relations are enshrined in political and socio-economic structures of inequality based on gender, race, ethnicity, class, sexual orientation, disability, age, etc. Also, bio-power, in the Foucauldian sense, as power used to manufacture consent through the control of knowledge and to govern people through the control of their bodies. 'A range of beliefs and practices around sexuality and reproduction – "proper" masculinity and femininity, child marriage, menarche rituals, menstruation practices, do's and don'ts around sex and childbearing especially among adolescents, people with disabilities or outside marriage, pregnancy and contraception, widowhood, gendered divisions of work and control over economic and other resources such as knowledge and information, heteronormative biases and discrimination, to name only some – provide ample evidence of such methods of obtaining compliance' (Sen et al., 2020, p. 2). In order to move forward with the realisation of SRHR, it is necessary to understand these power structures and relations and to find means to tackle them.

In sum, SRHR, unlike many other health-related domains, are not merely about health but encompass a wide range of social, political, and legal questions that are highly contentious. They touch on fundamental issues of social organisation, moral economy, and governance. This points both to the complexities of addressing SRHR issues and also to the fundamental need to do so in order to reduce social inequalities and ensure health and rights for all, including those most marginalised in society.

## Global Governance of SRHR

> Few global health organisations consider gender systematically in their policy-making and programming. They are impeded by their organisational cultures, political environments and characteristics of the issue. Among the barriers are entrenched, patriarchal practices; lack of training of professionals in these organisations to value gender analysis; conservative governments that view gender equality as a Western imposition; fear by government and global health officials that addressing gender will upset existing power relations; a conflation of gender with a concern for women and girls; and the complexity of the concept. Other barriers concern the proponents themselves: the absence of a cohesive community; differences among them on the nature of the problem and solutions, including which health issues to prioritize; and divergence on how to position the issue, particularly surrounding the use of instrumentalist, economics-oriented arguments.
>
> (Shawar & Shiffman, 2020, p. 9)

As argued earlier, SRHR has always been a contentious issue for global governance. In the early 1990s, a seeming high point was reached after strong global feminist mobilisation against more conservative elements who opposed the advancement of SRHR. The International Conference for Population and Development (ICPD) in 1994 was considered by many as a turning point in the SRHR landscape, where key actions were set in motion to enhance individual rights and improve the lives of women and girls, and by extension, their families and communities. The ambitious Programme of Action, which was adopted by consensus and later reaffirmed at ICPD +25, theoretically placed women and girls at the centre of development by supporting reproductive health and rights, as well as women's empowerment and gender equality, as cornerstones of population and development programmes. However, despite the "victory" of the adoption of the Programme of Action, there were limits both on what it contained and its potential for transformation into real action for women's SRHR. At the time of the negotiation of the Programme of Action, there was significant opposition, notably from the Vatican as well as from other states and international actors. The Programme of Action was thus accepted by consensus but with conditions placed on the language and terminology used, notably that reproductive rights did not include abortion or access to abortion care, any reference to couples in sexual relationships was not understood as the same sex, and "family" was considered a basic unit of society and founded in marriage (Corredor, 2019; United Nations Population Fund, 2004). There were also challenges in implementing the Plan of Action, resulting from a range of issues such as ideological opposition, lack of resources, or confusion over who was responsible for implementing the measures, with struggles documented both within and between different government ministries and between governments, international organisations, and non-governmental organisations (NGOs) (DeJong, 2000). So although the ICPD can be seen as a milestone for SRHR, the limitations that were evident at the time have persisted and, in some cases, amplified in the subsequent years. The resurgence of "anti-gender" movements at global and national levels (Denkovski et al., 2021; McEwen & Narayanaswamy, 2023) has contributed most recently to a real pushback against SRHR, and the limitations in the ICPD have become only more pronounced. This pushback was visible at the ICPD +25 and in the outcome document of the 68th session of the United Nations Commission on the Status of Women (CSW68) in 2024. We will return to this issue of pushback and its current implications later in the chapter.

### *The Shift from the MDGs to the SDGs*

The focus of SRH-related research, interventions, and indicators in the early 2000s was circumscribed, to a large extent, by the MDGs, where the SRH-related focus was on combating HIV and AIDS (Targets 6A and 6B) and improving maternal health (Target 5A), with the belated inclusion of access to universal reproductive health (Target 5B) in 2007. As we will argue in Chapter 5, this focus on HIV and AIDS has had important consequences for structuring international and regional politics and financing for SRHR. The subsequent adoption of the 2030 Agenda for Sustainable Development, with the stated aim of "leaving no one behind", has meant that the scope of SRHR intervention, with the Guttmacher-Lancet definition (Starrs et al., 2018) as the global guide, has rapidly expanded. Leaving no one behind has led to an increasing discourse on the SRHR needs of so-called "neglected groups" (Starrs et al., 2018). However, often a vague list of different people may fall into this category, demonstrating that there is no real understanding of who is neglected and why. Without a real understanding of the ways in which people are "neglected" or "made vulnerable", it is impossible to define real strategies to reach them and improve their SRHR.

### A Narrowing International Rights-Based Space

Global politics in the second decade of the 21st century has severely tested the optimism and buoyancy following the 1994 International Conference for Population Development in Cairo and the prospects of seeing SRHR realised for all. The increasingly hostile global political environment for rights-based SRH initiatives amidst the strengthening of right-wing and conservative forces antagonistic to gender equality on the political world stage has occurred alongside a rise in global economic inequalities. Within the international political arena, there has been a strengthening of so-called "anti-gender" movements (Denkovski et al., 2021; McEwen & Narayanaswamy, 2023), which has led a pushback against many of the gains made in promoting women's rights and gender equality, including in the domain of SRHR, and increasingly a regression in these rights. Anti-abortion politics have been central to these movements (Brooks et al., 2019; Erdman, 2016), and the ways in which anti-choice movements have managed to gain a foothold both in national and international political spaces have had important repercussions for the promotion of rights.

Anti-abortion politics in the United States have been central to these debates and have had a ripple effect globally. On 23 January 2017, the then President Trump issued *Protecting Life in Global Health Assistance* (PLGHA), an expansion of the Mexico City Policy, or "Global Gag Rule", last implemented under George W. Bush. PLGHA blocks US global health assistance to any foreign NGOs that perform abortions, except in cases of rape, incest, or threat to the life of the woman; provide counselling on or referrals for abortion; or lobby for the liberalisation of abortion law. The Global Gag Rule has been shown to have severe negative impacts on SRH care in many countries. McGovern et al. (2020) outline three crucial areas in which the PLGHA has had negative impacts. There is firstly decreased stakeholder coordination and a "chilling" of discussion related to SRHR, including the exclusion of many actors who have deep experience with these issues from discussions on SRHR at the national and international level, and a self-censorship in relation to speaking about abortion in policy fora. This has also led to a "ghettoization" of work on SRHR, which has become increasingly separated from general health systems in many countries. Secondly, the Act has led to reduced access to contraception for many women across the world, with attendant increases in unintended pregnancy and induced abortion. Finally, there have been negative outcomes beyond SRHR, including weakening of the overall health system functioning (McGovern et al., 2020).

In Southern Africa, where many countries already have weak public healthcare systems, the Global Gag Rule has a massive impact. A study by

Stanford University, for example, showed that when the rule was in place between 2001 and 2009, there was a dramatic rise in the number of induced abortions in Africa (Bendavid, Avila & Miller, 2011). Reduced SRH services also meant a reduction in access to contraceptives, which may have led to many unintended pregnancies and women turning to abortion as a result. The impacts of the Global Gag Rule have been widely felt both on women's access to safe abortion and to post-abortion care and in the wider perspective of SRH services provided by the same organisations which have been defunded under the terms of this rule. President Biden rescinded the Mexico City Policy shortly after taking office in January 2021, thus restoring the possibility of funding to many organisations working on issues of SRH around the world. However, the complexities of the rule and the fact that the Trump administration had reinforced restrictions mean that it could take months or even years for some organisations to regain their funding, if they regain it at all (Lieberman, 2021). Further, and perhaps even more worryingly, the negative effect of the policy on the ability to discuss abortion and related SRHR issues was a common finding of our research, where in most of the countries, informants spoke to us about the increasing difficulties of finding any public space to raise the issue of access to safe abortion (as we will discuss in more detail in Chapter 4). Whilst it has never been easy to discuss abortion in public or to place the issue on the political agenda, recent developments have led to increasing restrictions on public discussion, in some cases with official guidance or policy which limits this.

These and other efforts by highly sectarian and political forces culminated in 2022 with the overturning of the landmark *Roe v. Wade* ruling by the United States Supreme Court, ending the right to abortion for the past 50 years. Almost immediately, several states in the US enacted remarkably severe laws outlawing abortion – even in cases where the foetus is not viable and the mother's life is in danger. There is every indication that these groups intend to push for further restrictions in other areas of SRHR, such as access to contraception or the restriction of comprehensive sexuality education (CSE). While most countries in the Southern African Development Community (SADC) are largely viewed as progressive, there is concern around the "contagion" of these anti-gender movements, with influences from countries such as Uganda, which in 2023 passed a punitive *Anti-Homosexuality Bill,* and pressure for "Africanist" resistance against supposedly colonialist influence, lending weight to anti-gender movements and severely constraining space for the realisation of SRHR. What is fundamental to these initiatives is a concerted effort to detach rights from SRH – to deprive women of their bodily autonomy, diminish their hard-won gains in equality, and prevent access to every avenue of informed choice and independent action concerning their SRHR.

## The Southern African Context for SRHR

Across many countries in the region, marked successes in reducing infant and child mortality combined with high fertility amongst those of reproductive age mean that Africa has a very young age profile. This means that the current "youth bulge" of sexually active adolescents and young adults will grow still further and persist for decades as the generation of 0- to 14-year-olds also becomes sexually active. Against this background, the right to accessible, high-quality SRHR services is clearly fundamental to an individual's health and well-being over the life course. States in the Southern African region have made significant progress in improving some SRH indicators, most notably through reductions in maternal and child mortality and the drive towards the elimination of mother-to-child HIV transmission, increases in the numbers of people living with HIV initiated on treatment, and fewer deaths from AIDS-related illness. Progress, however, has been uneven, and in some cases, there has been a regression, with AGYW being disproportionately impacted.

AGYW in Southern Africa, as globally, are disproportionately burdened by poor SRHR and encounter numerous legal, economic, and social obstacles in accessing the SRH care they need and realising their rights. Prevailing harmful social norms and practices, restrictive legal contexts, and economic, social, and gender inequalities pose a major challenge to the attainment of a healthy sexual and reproductive life for all, particularly adolescent girls and young women. Of the AGYW who were newly infected with HIV globally in 2022, 80% live in SSA (UNAIDS, 2022). While global fertility rates have steeply declined, they still remain high in Africa, particularly amongst adolescents and young women. The United Nations Department of Economic and Social Affairs (UNDESA) projects that the region will continue to grow fast, with the population doubling in size by 2050, as compared to the population size in 2020; it is anticipated that the region will be the most populous globally in 2060.[1] These projections need to be considered against the fact that, compared to other regions, Africa had the highest unmet contraceptive need (43.7%) in 2020, and the adolescent birth rate was more than twice the world's average (102.1 vs 42.1 per 1000 women aged 15–19 years) (Poku et al., 2023).

Complications arising from unsafe abortion are a major cause of maternal morbidity and mortality in SSA, with highly restrictive abortion laws in most countries on the continent (Bearak et al., 2020). It is telling that the regulation of abortion, an issue that only impacts female reproductive bodies, is treated differently from all other types of health care, 'commonly regulated to varying degrees through the criminal law in addition to regulation under health-care law', including constitutions, reproductive health laws, health and medical ethics codes, guidelines, and judicial decisions (World Health Organisation, 2022, page 22). And unsafe abortion disproportionately impacts those who are the youngest and the poorest (Chae et al., 2017), since those with the financial means can access safe care privately or in neighbouring or nearby countries where abortion is legally available on request. Women are also disproportionately burdened by SGBV, with 1 in 3 women experiencing SGBV in their lifetime.[2] However, a higher proportion of women who have experienced violence continue to experience violence in lower income countries than in higher-income countries (Poku et al., 2023), where services for survivors of violence are frequently inadequate or non-existent. Other harmful practices include child marriage, where the global burden is increasingly shifting to SSA and where there are concerns that following ongoing conflict and human insecurity and climate change, this trend will continue (Corno et al., 2017; Malhotra & Elnakib, 2021; UNICEF, 2018). While child marriage is driven by a complex set of micro- and macro-level factors that differ widely across contexts, common to all contexts are the serious consequences for married girls, children of adolescent mothers, and society more broadly. Girl children are disproportionately affected by child marriage compared to boys (Gastón et al., 2019) and experience worse educational and health outcomes (Malhotra & Elnakib, 2021). These include low educational attainment, early and rapid repeat pregnancies, high fertility, and lower contraceptive use. Women married before 18 years of age also have a higher risk of sexual and physical intimate partner violence than those married when older (Kidman, 2017). Prevailing harmful social norms and practices, restrictive legal contexts, and economic, social, and gender inequalities pose a major challenge to the attainment of a healthy sexual and reproductive life for all, particularly AGYW.

## Country Case Studies

Our research, situated within this global and regional context, aims to provide a critical analysis of SRHR amongst AGYW in Southern Africa. We focus on five countries within the region: Madagascar, Mozambique, South Africa, Zambia, and Zimbabwe, where we have worked on various research projects with different (predominantly young) women. Although all of these countries obviously have very different political systems, legal structures, and economic conditions,[3] there are some elements which are comparable and shared across the national contexts and which have relevance for and impact on SRHR in each setting. The diversity of these case studies can also be used, we argue, to make more general claims about SRHR for AGYW in the Southern African region and more broadly.

SRHR cannot be discussed without recognising the reciprocal relationship between poverty and poor health – both of which are mutually reinforcing. SSA is the only region in the world that has not seen a decline in poverty levels. The five focus countries of our book are thus situated in a region where the world's poorest people live, and poverty is a critical contributor to poor health and a barrier to receiving health care. Rapid demographic growth, combined with a slowdown in economic growth and deepening of the public debt, have pushed countries in SSA further off track from ending extreme poverty by 2030 (SDG 1), and this will profoundly impact the attainment of SDGs 3 and 5. The COVID-19 pandemic has also deepened poverty and contributed to widening economic inequalities, and current economic conditions and recovery predictions are reportedly gloomier for the East and Southern African region than for other parts of SSA.[4] Macroeconomic stability in our five case study countries has been further threatened by high inflation (triple digits in Zimbabwe) and climate-related disasters, such as El-Nino-induced droughts in Zambia and South Africa and cyclones in Madagascar, Mozambique, and Zimbabwe.

The poor are disproportionately young, and live in large households in rural areas (Castañeda et al., 2018). Poor rural livelihoods are highly exposed and vulnerable to extreme weather events and disasters through climate change, and to a large extent, they are unable to absorb crop or livestock income losses and recover without national social protection programmes and investments in climate-resilient infrastructure. In 2019, cyclone Idai hit four of Mozambique's poorest provinces (Zambezia, Sofala, Tete, and Inhambane), and in 2021, the World Food Programme issued a warning that Southern Madagascar was on the brink of experiencing the world's first climate change-related famine. Poverty and periods of acute food insecurity create specific risks and vulnerabilities for girls and young women in terms of their SRHR (Crankshaw et al., 2021; Freedman et al., 2021). Of the five countries, Madagascar and Mozambique have the highest poverty levels, with 80.7% of the population in Madagascar living in extreme poverty and 64.6% in Mozambique.[5] Women tend to be more vulnerable to extreme poverty, as they spend more time on unpaid domestic responsibilities, have fewer assets, and have less access to remunerative employment than men. In Zambia, for example, women-headed households represent a third of the country's chronic poor, and upward mobility was found to be particularly challenging for this group, of whom the majority resides in rural areas (Shepherd et al., 2021). A historic bias in budgetary allocations to the urban and formal sector segments of Zambian society has meant that women and rural areas have long been disadvantaged by the political system and largely left to fend for themselves (Hinfelaar, 2021). In South Africa, which in 2023 had an employment rate of 31.9%, youth (15–34 years) and women of working age were disproportionately vulnerable to unemployment compared to older age groups and men, respectively.[6] In Zimbabwe, 38% of the population was living in extreme poverty in 2019, and there are indications that this figure is rapidly rising.[7]

Education is associated with higher living standards (Peet et al., 2015) and other benefits, such as a longer life expectancy; however, primary schooling is not sufficient to exit poverty (Castañeda et al., 2018). While enrolment is close to (and in some cases over 100% for primary education[8]) and reaches gender parity in all five countries, country data presents a more sombre picture of young people's ability to transition to secondary and tertiary education. Aside from South Africa, educational trajectories tend to end for most young people on completion of primary education, and thus the prospects of increasing their chances of formal sector employment through secondary schooling or advancing to tertiary education are low.[9] Opportunity costs related to studying, and early marriage or pregnancy act as important deterrent for enrolment and completion of secondary education (Arias et al., 2019). Expanded and equitable access to secondary education for both genders and children from poor(er) households requires substantial public investment to keep pace with the region's growing primary education completion rates and youthful population. In all countries, except South Africa, the African Development Bank reported that in 2022, around 40% of the population was below the age of 15, and around 20% between the ages of 15 and 24 years.

Young people's access to health services, when they need them, is severely constrained for multiple reasons, including a critical shortage of skilled health workforce and inequitable distribution of facilities and health workers in Madagascar, Mozambique, South Africa, Zambia, and Zimbabwe.[10] In Mozambique, there are only 8.5 medical doctors and 47.3 nurses and midwives available per 100,000 people. In Zambia, there are 9.3 doctors and 93.1 nurses/midwives per 100,000 people; in Madagascar, there are 18.1 and 29.8 per 100,000 people, respectively; and in Zimbabwe, there are 22 doctors and 193.5 nurses/midwives. South Africa is the exception, with 75.3 doctors per 100,000 people.[11] While new health professionals are being trained, the financial capability of countries[12] to pay the wage bill and fill the human resource gaps, even partially, forms a major bottleneck to meeting the health needs of young people and their families in Madagascar, Mozambique, South Africa, Zambia, and Zimbabwe – and particularly in the rural areas that are typically under-resourced and underserved.

In 2013, all five countries committed to scaling up the provision of youth-friendly SRH services, improving independent access to these services for adolescents and young people, and reaching most adolescents before puberty with age-appropriate CSE during primary school education (UNESCO, 2013). By signing the Eastern and Southern Africa Ministerial Commitment on CSE and Youth Friendly SRH Services, the country's Ministers of Health and Education pledged to reduce new HIV infections and unintended pregnancies among adolescents and young people and eliminate child marriage and gender-based violence by 2020. South Africa, Mozambique, Zambia, and Zimbabwe recently renewed their commitments, but substantial gaps in access to information and services among adolescents and young people remain in the region. Teenage pregnancies are high in all case study countries (Ayalew et al., 2022; Neal et al., 2020). The restricted movement and closure of workspaces and schools during the various lockdowns during the COVID-19 pandemic have further contributed to increasing levels of SGBV and early and unintended pregnancies in all these countries. It is unclear whether country roadmaps to 2030 will be sufficient to overcome some of the key challenges to implementation, which include the need for multisectoral action amongst the very different ministry mandates of health and education, ideological resistance to CSE, and, with the exception of South Africa, a continued punitive legal and policy environment for SRHR (Machawira et al., 2020; Watson et al., 2021). And even in South Africa, implementation challenges persist.

Legal and regulatory frameworks raise significant barriers for young people in obtaining full and equal access to health information, education, and services, and restrictions become even more pronounced when it pertains to their SRHR for all the reasons discussed above. For example, AGYW may require parental or spousal consent before being able to access SRH services based on their age or marital status. Some of the age of consent requirements in SRHR service provision have their origins in foreign laws, which include a 1920 French colonial framework which was enacted in Madagascar and which prohibited the distribution of contraception to youth or married women without parental or spousal consent. With the passage of Law No. 90-030 in 1990, family planning and contraception in Madagascar received a more positive connotation and were recognised as an essential component in advancing the country's social and economic development. In 2017, a new Reproductive Health and Family Planning law was passed, facilitating people's access to contraception, regardless of age or marital status, and lifting previous consent requirements. However, the lifting of the requirement for consent for young women under the age of 18 is still not widely known amongst health workers in the country (Freedman et al., 2021). Indeed, in all case study countries, with perhaps the exception of South Africa which has stand alone and explicit contraceptive guidelines (South African Department of Health. 2012), lack of clarity around, and lack of harmonisation in laws and policies on age of consent consigns young people's requests to the personal discretion of healthcare providers when accessing contraceptive or other SRHR services, such as HIV testing and screening for STIs. In the absence of clarity, the minimum age of consent to sexual intercourse, when stated in the law, tends to serve as a surrogate. In the case of Zambia, this implies that a young person below the age of 16 will be denied access to a service without parental consent, and our country study confirmed this practice for contraceptive services at the facility level. Nonetheless, the Zambia Family Planning Guidelines and Protocols state the following: 'facilitate access, especially for young girls, to all types of services dealing with reproductive health concerns, and specifically family planning without consent of spouse, parents/guardians or relatives as allowed by current legislation' (Government of the Republic of Zambia, 2006, p. 2). The legal provision of abortion care in Zambia is upheld against the consent age for a medical or surgical procedure, which means that young people below the age of 18 cannot procure a legal abortion without the consent of their parents. To guarantee young people's right to access information, education, and services, international bodies such as the UNFPA and WHO recommend to establish the age of consent to seek and receive medical treatment without parental consent at 12 years of age and access to information on SRHR and services to be made available from 10 years of age (World Health Organisation, 2018a). Countries are further advised to enact legislation which distinguishes medical treatment from surgical operations with a view to more clearly differentiating between medical treatment that a minor can access at the age of 12 without parental consent and major medical procedures for which the minor first requires the consent of a parent or guardian.

The Maputo Protocol enshrines women's right to access comprehensive reproductive health care services and information on contraception and safe abortion care without discrimination. It also obliges state parties to create the legal, economic, and social conditions that enable women to exercise their sexual and reproductive rights with regard to family planning/contraception and safe abortion. It is the main legal instrument for the protection of rights for girls and women in terms of economic and political empowerment, health, and well-being, and the first pan-African treaty to explicitly recognise abortion as a human right under specific circumstances. These circumstances include sexual assault, rape, and incest and in cases where a continued pregnancy endangers the mental and physical health of the mother, the life of the mother, or the life of the foetus (art 14.2c.). With the exception of Botswana, Malawi, and Madagascar, all SADC Member states have both signed and ratified the Maputo Protocol (Botswana has neither signed nor ratified, Madagascar has signed but not ratified, and Malawi has ratified but not signed). South Africa and Mozambique have the most liberal TOP laws of all the SADC member states, with abortion being allowed within gestational limits on request. In Zambia, the 1972 TOP Act, amended in 1994, stipulates that, 'In determining whether the continuance of a pregnancy would involve such risk as is mentioned in paragraph (a) of subsection (1), *account may be taken of the pregnant woman's actual or reasonably foreseeable environment* or of her age (authors own emphasis)'. This has widely been interpreted in the academic literature that Zambia allows TOPs on socioeconomic grounds (Fetters et al., 2017; Haaland et al., 2019), and this is reinforced in the Zambian MoH 2017 Standards and Guidelines for Comprehensive Abortion Care which states that in 'assess(ing) the environment the provider may consider the situation of the woman as regards: Medical, Economic situation, Social/cultural circumstance, Religious etc' (Government of the Republic of Zambia., 2017, p 24).

In Zimbabwe, abortion is not permitted on request or on socioeconomic grounds. However, abortion is allowed under conditions of foetal impairment, rape, and incest to preserve the physical health or life of the woman. There are additional provisions for pregnancies occurring amongst people living with mental disabilities and people living with HIV. In Mozambique and Zambia, parental consent of minors is required before a minor can access an abortion, which may pose a significant barrier to a young person who doesn't wish for their parent to know about a pregnancy. In South Africa, parental and spousal consent are explicitly stated as not required. In Zimbabwe, parental consent for minors and judicial authorisation for minors are also explicitly stated as not required. Abortion is prohibited in all circumstances in Madagascar. Attempts to modify Article 317 of the penal code in Madagascar and expand the grounds for a legal abortion in 2022 were unsuccessful, largely due to organised lobbying by religious leaders. The regulation of abortions through criminal law differs from the regulation of other health procedures, and this holds serious implications for the health and rights of women and girls as well as for health service providers who risk criminal sanctions (including imprisonment) if they are convicted of having helped to provide an abortion. The stigma associated with seeking and providing abortions when the procedure is criminalised can cause trained health providers to act more cautiously or refuse care and increase women and girls' recourse to unsafe abortions (World Health Organisation, 2022). It may also delay or discourage women and girls from accessing post-abortion care when these services are legally and widely available to them (ibid.).

### *Some Ethical Considerations*

Whilst there are minimum ethical standards that are required for all research that involves human subjects, there are additional ethical considerations for research that is conducted among minors (<18 years of age) as well as marginalised, hard-to-reach and/or criminalised populations (e.g. refugees or sex workers) due to their legal minority and/or precarious and vulnerable positions in which the research can place them when operating in an illegal context. The different research projects on which this book is based involved navigating particular interlocking and overlapping conceptual, methodological, and ethical considerations amongst young refugee women (Crankshaw and Mutambara, 2024), and in other cases, our research included populations who were minors who were also engaged in criminalised behaviours (e.g. selling sex, homosexuality, and illegal substance use) and/or criminalised procedures (induced abortions). In the case of research amongst minors, institutional review boards or research ethics committees require parental written consent and adolescent assent for participation in any research. However, obtaining parental consent for minors who are engaged in criminalised behaviours (selling sex/injecting drug use/homosexuality) is not an option for many of these adolescents whose activities are unknown to the family or who are estranged from their family or orphaned. An exception to the requirement of parental consent for adolescents aged 16 years and above is possible if adolescents can be considered "emancipated minors". Such will be the case for adolescents who themselves are parents or expecting parents, married or living in a marital union, and/or are living separate or apart from their parents. If such was the case in our respective research, adolescents were asked to sign a written informed consent form with no requirements for parental consent. Institutional and in country ethics approvals were, respectively, obtained for all the research studies and as appropriate.

An additional layer of ethical complexity within our research projects was the inclusion of minors who self-identified as being involved in "sex work". According to UN definitions of sex work (UNAIDS, 2002), anyone 'who receives money or goods in exchange for sexual services, either regularly or occasionally' is considered to be a sex worker. However, if they are under 18 years of age, they are considered to be a sexually exploited child under Article 34 of the Convention on the Rights of the Child (World Health Organisation, 2015). This has had the effect of rendering young women <18 years who are engaged in selling sex largely invisible in research, with researchers deterred by the ethical complexities of including them in the research and, in some countries, mandatory reporting requirements in place, resulting in a lack of understanding of their unique vulnerabilities and needs (Crankshaw et al., 2021; Silverman, 2011). Our intersectional approach views age as a key social categorisation within the matrices of inequality and vulnerability. However, the above-imposed definitions sometimes provided us with difficulties in obtaining ethical approval to conduct the research. Therefore, we adopted slightly different strategies in the various country contexts according to national and international ethical norms regarding this question. For this reason, since our research in Zimbabwe, Mozambique, and Zambia specifically included young people who self-identified as selling sex and/or persons of diverse gender identity and sexual orientations, we only recruited older adolescents 16–24 years since adolescents who are 16 and 17 years are considered mature minors. This is in keeping with the Convention on the Rights of the Child's consideration of the concept of children's evolving capacities (Articles 5 and 14). In addition, only those within this age group of adolescents can legally gain the status of emancipated minors. The research in Madagascar recruited adolescents from the general population, and therefore those aged 15–24 years were included in the research. In South Africa, we only recruited migrant and refugee women aged 18–24 years due to language and logistical difficulties in obtaining parental consent. In all cases where parental consent was required, this was only obtained with prior permission from the adolescent. In order to safeguard young people's privacy, we explained to their parents/guardians that the focus of the study was on young people *in general* and on their SRH experiences, concerns, and needs.

Depending on the country context, criminalisation laws can be enforced punitively and carry mandatory reporting requirements for researchers who engage with these populations, thereby exposing a research participant to potential harm. In determining our ethical obligation if a minor was involved in sexual practices that may be considered statutory rape or selling sex, we acted in the best interest of the child embedded in the specific country setting. According to the World Health Organisation (2018b), in acting in the best interests of the child, the researcher must 'identify what risks a child could be exposed to if an action is taken versus if an action is not taken'. Reporting statutory rape that is revealed in the course of research has the very real potential to bring harm to study participants, especially in the study country contexts which do not have strong welfare support mechanisms or where the authorities tend to act punitively rather than supportive in contexts where selling sex is illegal and highly stigmatised. Additionally, because some cultures accept or encourage young women to form relationships with older men, as is the case with some of our study countries, reporting these cases may violate cultural norms and bring distress to a young woman, her partner, and often family members who are frequently complicit in these pairings. We view the above dynamics very seriously and had senior and experienced researchers leading the research at the country level, as well as highly trained broader research teams supporting them. Rather than undertaking to report statutory rape, we received permission from the in country ethics committees to work with local NGOs and outreach programmes to provide minors with support – with the consent or at the request of the minor involved. As is standard good practice for all research and a requirement by some research ethics committees, strong referral pathways for a wide range of support for participants were established prior to the fieldwork commencing, and participants were referred as needed. This involved working closely with in country research partners in identifying and mapping the local organisations which offered the relevant services at no cost to participants.

The situation wherein minors are engaged in sexual economic exchanges is a reality across the region and was raised in all our study settings. Throughout the various research projects, we engaged in ongoing consultation with ethico-legal experts within our academic networks to, as far as possible, anticipate and plan for any potential ethical/legal issues arising in the course of the fieldwork, as well as how to best navigate the reality that sometimes behaving ethically in one's research practice means not reporting illegal behaviours to authorities (Strode & Slack, 2020). Although researchers can prepare and institute as many safeguards as possible ahead of embarking on fieldwork, the reality is that it is impossible to predict what ethical dilemmas or "ethically important moments" may arise in the field or how these should be dealt with (Guillemin & Gillam, 2004, p. 262). This dynamism is especially experienced in qualitative research, which by its very design is not predetermined and provides opportunity for new and emerging understandings. For this reason, the concept of reflexivity has been identified as a useful tool to ensure "ethics in practice" or "microethics", which should occur over and above formal or "procedural ethics", which involves obtaining the necessary study approvals from research ethics committees (Guillemin & Gillam, 2004). A reflexive approach creates the space for the researcher to acknowledge and be sensitised to the day-to-day ethical tensions that may arise in the course of research and be more prepared to deal with them (Guillemin & Gillam, 2004). In this way, being reflexive can be an enabling tool towards ethical practice, which can be especially useful in research that focuses on complex transnational issues (Block et al. 2012).

## Migration and Gender in Southern Africa

One of the case studies for the book focuses on women refugees in South Africa. Our interest in including this case study was to understand another intersecting structure of inequality: that related to citizenship and nationality status. Given the scale of intra-regional migration in the Southern African region, this axis of inequality cannot be ignored when carrying out intersectional analysis.

Intra-regional migration has been a continuous feature of the regional landscape in Southern Africa since the mid-19th century, and there are currently an estimated 4.5 million migrants in the region, a figure which has remained relatively stable since the 1990s (Crush et al., 2017). Historically, migration flows largely consisted of male labour migrants in search of work opportunities in the mining and agricultural industries. However, increasingly feminised migration patterns have been documented in the region (Fleury, 2016). In 2013, 44% of the 4 million migrants recorded in the region were female, and 20% were below the age of 19 years (Pophiwa, 2014). With continued conflict, civil unrest, and economic instability on the African continent, migration to and within the Southern African region is characterised by increasing diversity, with migration for multiple reasons – commerce, employment, family and marriage migration, and asylum seekers and refugees.

In countries of destination, such as South Africa, gendered inequalities and structures of violence also shape the experiences of women migrants and refugees, who may experience greater difficulty in accessing asylum procedures or gaining legal residence status or work permits. In many cases, their residence status is tied to that of a male partner, which creates problems of legal dependence (Freedman et al., 2020). Further, women might find access to formal labour markets more difficult and can be caught in informal, exploitative employment relations. For many migrant women, transactional sexual relationships may be an important way of being able to cross borders, gain protection, and earn a livelihood. In the Southern African region, the interactions between migration and sex work have been underexplored (Richter et al., 2014), including the health implications of these interactions. Similarly, there is very little research which explores migrant and refugee women's involvement in transactional sexual relationships, the factors that lead to these types of relationships, or the consequences for the women involved. The experiences of women migrants are mediated by other intersecting social identities, such as sexual orientation, class, race, nationality, and age.

South Africa has for many years been a country of destination for asylum seekers and refugees from across the Southern African region. In 2020, the United Nations High Commission for Refugees (UNHCR) estimated that there were over 250,000 asylum seekers and refugees in South Africa, of whom most were asylum seekers awaiting a decision on their claims. Many of these asylum seekers and refugees originate from other African countries, particularly the Democratic Republic of the Congo, Ethiopia, Somalia, Burundi, Congo, or Zimbabwe. As elsewhere in the world, there is a gender imbalance in the numbers of asylum seekers in South Africa, with men generally making up the majority of asylum claimants. In 2015, men represented 67% of asylum claimants and women only 33% (Crush et al. 2017). These figures should not, however, be interpreted as meaning that women suffer less violence and persecution and are thus less in need of refugee protection.

Our case study on women refugees thus enriches our understandings of situated intersectional vulnerabilities and the negative SRHR outcomes associated with them.

## Plan of the Book

In the following chapters, we first take a theoretical look at the concept of vulnerability and what it means to be made vulnerable in the context of SRHR. We argue for an understanding of vulnerability based on a situated intersectional approach and not on a "vulnerable groups" approach, and we discuss the implications of this for thinking about SRHR policies and programmes. We then go on in subsequent chapters to discuss specific areas of SRHR that adopt this situated intersectional approach. Chapter 3 examines the ways in which young women are involved in sexual-economic exchanges and the implications of the dominance of the categorisations of "sex work" and "transactional sex" in international policies and interventions. Chapter 4 returns to the way in which the HIV response has structured policies and programmes on SRHR and argues for a broadening of the focus in order to ensure reaching the most marginalised and ensuring SRHR for all, moving beyond an approach based on risk to one based on rights. And then Chapter 5 comes back to the ever present and fundamental attack on SRHR posed by the prevalence of SGBV. Finally, in Chapter 6, we conclude by bringing together the analysis presented in the previous chapters to show what our research could bring to both research and policy agendas going forward, in view of deepening climate-related vulnerabilities in the future.

## Notes

1 UNDESA, 2021. Global Population Growth and Sustainable Development. UNDESA/POP/2021/TR/NO. 2.
2 World Health Organisation, 2022.
3 Madagascar, Mozambique and Zambia are classified as low-income countries (LIC) by the World Bank – Zambia was previously classified as a lower middle-income country (LMIC) but in 2023 re-classified as an LIC due to the deterioration of Gross National Income per capita estimates recorded in 2021. Zimbabwe was previously classified as an LIC but in 2020 reclassified as an LMIC. South Africa is classified as an upper middle income country.
4 Source: World Bank, 2023. https://www-worldbank-org.vu-nl.idm.oclc.org/en/region/afr/overview
5 World Bank. Poverty and equity brief, African Eastern and Southern. Madagascar. Mozambique. April 2023.
6 https://www.gov.za/news/media-statements/statistics-south-africa-quarterly-labour-force-survey-quarter-three-2023-14
7 World Bank. Poverty & Equity Brief: Zimbabwe. Africa Eastern & Southern, October 2021.
8 Gross enrolment ratios in primary education are over a 100% in Mozambique and South Africa. Enrolment can exceed 100% due to the inclusion of over-aged and under-aged pupils because of early or late entrants, and grade repetition.
9 Gross enrolment ratio in secondary education, presented as an aggregate for the period 2011–2021, is particularly low in Madagascar (34.6%) and Mozambique (35.4%). The ratio is 52.4% in Zimbabwe, South Africa 102.6%, while data for this period was not available on Zambia. Source: African Development Bank Group Repository, social data. https://dataportal.opendataforafrica.org/Social_Data_Country
10 WHO recommends a minimum threshold of 2.3 skilled health workers per 1000 people (doctors, nurses and midwives) in its Road map for scaling up the human resources for health for improved health service delivery in the African region 2012–2025.
11 AFDB aggregate data 2010-2019. Data on nurses and midwives is not available from South Africa.
12 Government health expenditure as a percentage of the gross domestic product was reported to be 3.7% in 2019 in Madagascar, 5.3% Zambia, 7.7% in Zimbabwe, 7.8% Mozambique, and 9.1% in South Africa. Source: AFDB 2019 data.

## References


Arias, O., Evans, D. K., & Santos, I. (2019). *The skills balancing act in Sub-Saharan Africa: Investing in skills for productivity, inclusivity, and adaptability*. World Bank Publications.

Ayalew, H. G., Liyew, A. M., Tessema, Z. T., Worku, M. G., Tesema, G. A., Alamneh, T. S., Teshale, A. B., Yeshaw, Y., & Alem, A. Z. (2022). Prevalence and factors associated with unintended pregnancy among adolescent girls and young women in sub-Saharan Africa, a multilevel analysis. *BMC Womens Health, 22*(1), 464.

Bearak, J., Popinchalk, A., Ganatra, B., Moller, A. B., Tunçalp, Ö, Beavin, C., Kwok, L., & Alkema, L. (2020). Unintended pregnancy and abortion by income, region, and the legal status of abortion: Estimates from a comprehensive model for 1990–2019. *The Lancet Global Health, 8*(9), e1152–e1161.

Bendavid, E., Avila, P., & Miller, G. (2011). United States aid policy and induced abortion in sub-Saharan Africa. *Bulletin of the World Health Organisation*, *89*(12), 873–880.

Block, K., Warr, D., Gibbs, L., & Riggs, E. (2012). Addressing ethical and methodological challenges in research with refugee-background young people: Reflections from the field. *Journal of Refugee Studies*, *26*(1), 69–87.

Brooks, N., Bendavid, E., & Miller, G. (2019). USA aid Policy and induced abortion in sub-Saharan Africa: An analysis of the Mexico City policy. *The Lancet Global Health*, *7*(8), e1046–e1053.

Castañeda, A., Doan, D., Newhouse, D., Nguyen, M. C., Uematsu, H., & Azevedo, J. P. (2018). A new profile of the global poor. *World Development*, *101*, 250–267.

Chae, S., Desai, S., Crowell, M., Sedgh, G., & Singh, S. (2017). Characteristics of women obtaining induced abortions in selected low-and middle-income countries. *PloS One*, *12*(3), e0172976.

Corno, L., Hildebrandt, N., & Voena, A. (2017). *Age of marriage, weather shocks, and the direction of marriage payments*. Working Paper 23604. National Bureau of Economic Research.

Corredor, E. S. (2019). Unpacking "gender ideology" and the global right's antigender countermovement. *Journal of Women in Culture and Society*, *44*(3), 613–638.

Crankshaw, T. L., Chareka, S., Zambezi, P., & Poku, N. K. (2021). Age matters: Determinants of sexual and reproductive health vulnerabilities amongst young women who sell sex (16–24 years) in Zimbabwe. *Social Science & Medicine*, *270*, 113597.

Crankshaw, T. L., & Mutambara, M. (2024). Conducting sexual and reproductive health and rights research amongst refugee women in Sub Saharan Africa: Some ethical and methodological considerations. In: Jane Freedman and Glenda Santana de Andrade (Eds.), *Research handbook on asylum and refugee policy*, Edward Elgar.

Crush, J., Dodson, B., Williams, V., & Tevara, D. (2017). Harnessing migration for inclusive growth and development in Southern Africa (pp. i–64). Vienna: International Centre for Migration Policy Development and Waterloo, ON: Southern African Migration Programme.

DeJong, J. (2000). The role and limitations of the Cairo international conference on population and development. *Social Science & Medicine*, *51*(6), 941–953.

Denkovski, D., Bernarding, N., & Lunz, K. (2021). Power Over Rights. *Understanding and countering the transnational anti-gender movement Volume I.*

Erdman, J. N. (2016). The politics of global abortion rights. *The Brown Journal of World Affairs*, *22*(2), 39–57.

Fetters, T., Samandari, G., Djemo, P., Vwallika, B., & Mupeta, S. (2017). Moving from legality to reality: How medical abortion methods were introduced with implementation science in Zambia. *Reproductive Health*, *14*, 1–11.

Fleury, A., 2016. *Understanding women and migration: a literature review*. KNOMAD working paper 8. Global Knowledge Partnerships on Migration and Development (KNOMAD).

Freedman, J., Crankshaw, T. L., & Mutambara, V. M. (2020). Sexual and reproductive health of asylum seeking and refugee women in South Africa. *Sexual and Reproductive Health Matters*, *28*(1), 324–334.

Freedman, J., Rakotoarindrasata, M., & de Dieu Randrianasolorivo, J. (2021). Analysing the economies of transactional sex amongst young people: Case study of Madagascar. *World Development*, *138*, 105289.

Gastón, C. M., Misunas, C., & Cappa, C. (2019). Child marriage among boys: A global overview of available data. *Vulnerable Children and Youth Studies*, *14*(3), 219–28. https://doi.org/10.1080/17450128.2019.1566584.

Government of the Republic of Zambia (2006). *Family planning guidelines and protocols*. Ministry of Health.
Government of the Republic of Zambia (2017). *Standards and guidelines for comprehensive abortion care in Zambia*. Ministry of Health.
Guillemin, M., & Gillam, L. (2004). Ethics, reflexivity, and "ethically important moments" in research. *Qualitative Inquiry*, *10*(2), 261–280.
Haaland, M. E., Haukanes, H., Zulu, J. M., Moland, K. M., Michelo, C., Munakampe, M. N., & Blystad, A. (2019). Shaping the abortion policy–competing discourses on the Zambian termination of pregnancy act. *International Journal for Equity in Health*, *18*(1), 1–11.
Hinfelaar, M. (2021). The political economy of poverty dynamics in Zambia. Working paper. www.chronicpovertynetwork.org
Kidman, R. (2017). Child marriage and intimate partner violence: A comparative study of 34 countries. *International Journal of Epidemiology*, *46*(2), 662–75.
Lieberman, A. (2021). Biden repeals the 'Global gag rule,'but next steps will be 'Huge undertaking.' *Devex*. Accessed January 28, 2021.
Machawira, P., Castle, C., & Herat, J. (2020). Progress and challenges with comprehensive sexuality education. What does this mean for HIV prevention in the region? In K. Govender, & N. K. Poku (Eds.), *Preventing HIV among young people in Southern and Eastern Africa: Emerging evidence and intervention strategies* (pp. 262–279). Routledge.
Malhotra, A., & Elnakib, S. (2021). *Evolution in the evidence base on child marriage 2000-2019*. UNFPA-UNICEF Global Programme to End Child Marriage.
McEwen, H., & Narayanaswamy, L. (2023). *The international anti-gender movement: Understanding the rise of anti-gender discourses in the context of development, human rights and social protection* (No. 2023-06). UNRISD Working Paper.
McGovern, T., Schaaf, M., Battistini, E., Maistrellis, E., Gibb, K., & Casey, S. E. (2020). From bad to worse: Global governance of abortion and the global gag rule. *Sexual and Reproductive Health Matters*, *28*(3), 54–63.
Morgan, L. M., & Roberts, E. F. (2012). Reproductive governance in Latin America. *Anthropology & Medicine*, *19*(2), 241–254.
Neal, S., Channon, A. A., Chandra-Mouli, V., & Madise, N. (2020). Trends in adolescent first births in sub-Saharan Africa: A tale of increasing inequity? *International Journal for Equity in Health*, *19*, 1–11.
Peet, E. D., Fink, G., & Fawzi, W. (2015). Returns to education in developing countries: Evidence from the living standards and measurement study surveys. *Economics of Education Review*, *49*, 69–90.
Poku, N. K., Strauss, M., Crankshaw, T. L., & Chareka, S. (2023). *Sexual and reproductive health and rights in East and Southern Africa*. Health Economics and HIV and AIDS Research Division, University of KwaZulu-Natal.
Pophiwa, N. (2014). The drivers and outcomes of feminization of migration in Africa, Pambazuka News, 26 June 2014, https://www.pambazuka.org/gender-minorities/drivers-and-outcomes-feminization-migration-africa.
Richter, M., Chersich, M. F., Vearey, J., Sartorius, B., Temmerman, M., & Luchters, S. (2014). Migration status, work conditions and health utilization of female sex workers in three South African cities. *Journal of Immigrant and Minority Health*, *16*, 7–17.
Sen, G., Iyer, A., Chattopadhyay, S., & Khosla, R. (2020). When accountability meets power: Realizing sexual and reproductive health and rights. *International Journal of Equity in Health*, 19, 111. https://doi.org/10.1186/s12939-020-01221-4.
Sen, G., Kismödi, E., & Knutsson, A. (2019). Moving the ICPD agenda forward: Challenging the backlash. *Sexual and Reproductive Health Matters*, *27*(1), 319–322.

Shawar, Y. R., & Shiffman, J. (2020). Political challenges to prioritizing gender in global health organisations. *Journal of Global Health, 10*(1).

Shepherd, A., Bond, V., Bwalya, C., Bwalya, R., Chapoto, A., da Corta, L., Diwaker, V., Eichsteller, M., Gwanu, L., Lubungu, M., Mwamba, M., Ndubani, P., Simbaya, J., & Subakany, M. (2021). Zambia poverty dynamics. National Report. Chronic Poverty Advisory Network, Overseas Development Institute, London. https://dl.orangedox.com/9bu9JXybje3v087SWK

Silverman, J. G. (2011). Adolescent female sex workers: invisibility, violence and HIV. *Archives of Disease in Childhood, 96*(5), 478–481.

South African Department of Health. (2012). The South African National Contraception Clinical Guidelines. Available at: https://www.gov.za/sites/default/files/gcis_document/201409/contraceptionclinicalguidelines28jan2013-2.pdf

Starrs, A. M., Ezeh, A. C., Barker, G., Basu, A., Bertrand, J. T., Blum, R., & Ashford, L. S. (2018). Accelerate progress—Sexual and reproductive health and rights for all: Report of the Guttmacher–Lancet Commission. *The Lancet, 391*(10140), 2642–2692.

Strode, A. E., & Slack, C. M. (2020). Three billboards to support ethical-legal adolescent HIV prevention research in Eastern and Southern Africa. In K. Govender, & N. K. Poku (Eds.), *Preventing HIV among young people in Southern and Eastern Africa: Emerging evidence and intervention strategies* (pp. 92–109). Routledge.

UNAIDS. (2002). *Technical update sex work and HIV/AIDS.* Geneva. Joint United Nations Programme on HIV/AIDS. https://www.unaids.org/en/resources/documents/2002/20020704_jc705-sexwork-tu_en.pdf

UNAIDS. (2022). *In danger: UNAIDS global AIDS update 2022.* Geneva: Joint United Nations Programme on HIV/AIDS.

UNESCO. (2013). Eastern and Southern Africa Ministerial commitment on comprehensive sexuality education and sexual and reproductive health services for adolescents and young people.

United Nations General Assembly. (2006). United Nations General Assembly Resolution A/RES/60/1.

United Nations General Assembly. (2015). United Nations General Assembly Resolution A/RES/65/1.

United Nations Population Fund. (2004). Programme of Action, adopted at the International Conference for Population and Development, Cairo, 5–13 September 1994.

UNICEF. 2018. Child Marriage: Latest trends and future prospects.

Watson, K., Akwara, E., Machawira, P., Bakaroudis, M., Tallarico, R., & Chandra-Mouli, V. (2021). The East and Southern Africa Ministerial Commitment: A review of progress toward fulfilling young people's sexual and reproductive health and rights (2013–2018). *Sexual and Reproductive Health Matters, 29*(1), 261–286.

World Health Organisation. (2015). *Technical brief: HIV and young people who sell sex.* Geneva: World Health Organisation. https://www.who.int/publications/i/item/WHO-HIV-2015.7

World Health Organisation. (2018a). *Recommendations on adolescent sexual and reproductive health and rights, 2018.*

World Health Organisation. (2018b). *Guidance on ethical considerations in planning and reviewing research studies on sexual and reproductive health in adolescents.*

World Health Organisation (2022). *Abortion care guideline.* Geneva: World Health Organisation

# 2 UNDERSTANDING AND IDENTIFYING VULNERABILITY IN SRHR RESEARCH AND POLICY

## Introduction

Vulnerability is a term which has become somewhat ubiquitous when considering various SRHR issues. However, the ways in which this concept has been utilised and applied to SRHR policies and programmes can be questioned. We mentioned in the introduction that one of the central research projects on which this book is based originated in an approach that identified "key populations" as groups which were intrinsically or essentially vulnerable to HIV (and thus poor SRHR), but that we came to the realisation that this group-based approach did not allow us to understand both differences within "key populations" nor similarities between members of these "key populations" and others outside of the group. This led us to question the group-based definition of vulnerability and, thus, to try and define and understand vulnerabilities in a different way. In this chapter, we turn to the work of Martha Fineman and her definitions of vulnerability within a broader SRHR lens and to the critiques of this work in order to try and provide a more adequate understanding of what vulnerability is and how and why young people may be placed in situations of vulnerability to poor SRHR. We then outline how this definition and approach could be useful for advancing knowledge and policymaking on SRHR. We start with a short overview of existing legal and political frameworks for SRHR, both internationally and regionally, in order to understand the context within which these debates over vulnerability and SRHR are taking place.

## Political and Legal Frameworks for SRHR

The Protocol to the African Charter on Human and People's Rights on the Rights of Women in Africa – more commonly known as the "Maputo Protocol" based

DOI: 10.4324/9781003414698-2

on the city in Mozambique where it was signed in 2003 – is a continental human rights treaty of the African Union. The Maputo Protocol enshrines women's right to access comprehensive reproductive health care services and information on contraception and safe abortion without discrimination. The Maputo Protocol is a legally binding instrument, and with the exception of Madagascar, Malawi, and Botswana,[1] all SADC Member States have signed and ratified the Maputo Protocol. In 2006, the AU Heads of State adopted a second policy framework which focused specifically on sexual and reproductive health: the Continental Policy Framework on Sexual and Reproductive Health and Rights (CPF). The purpose of this framework is to provide guidance to national governments in implementing the ICPD Plan of Action and in developing SRHR policies. The policy statement clearly lays out the need for a Continent-wide mainstreaming of reproductive health programmes and the harmonisation of reproductive health issues into development initiatives at all levels. The policy framework calls for mainstreaming[2] SRHR in primary health care and mainstreaming gender in all development programmes of member states. It also calls for the implementation of the Abuja declaration, which aims to increase resources for the health sector and improve access to services. Preceded by the Maputo Plan of Action 2007–2015, which operationalises the CPF, the revised Maputo Plan of Action 2016–2030 aims to ensure universal access to comprehensive sexual and reproductive health services in Africa beyond 2015. Most recently, in May 2023, the Africa Centres for Disease Control and Prevention (Africa CDC) officially launched its Reproductive Health Strategy Priorities 2022–2026 to improve maternal and reproductive health in Africa and to make progress towards reducing high levels of maternal mortality amongst the sovereign states that make up the AU. This strategy is aimed at supporting and accelerating the monitoring of the MPoA 2016–2030 and is driven by the Reproductive Health Unit of the Africa CDC.

The Southern African Development Community (SADC), which is one of the eight Regional Economic Communities in the AU, has normative frameworks in place that contain commitments to gender equality and the rights of adolescent girls and women. One such framework is the 'Regional Strategy for Sexual and Reproductive Health and Rights (2019–2030) in the SADC region',[3] which provides the scaffolding for the 16 Member States to address SRHR in the region. The strategy is also accompanied by a multi-sectoral scorecard to support implementation. There is a second related strategy that is also linked to our book focus and which therefore needs mentioning; this is the 'Regional Strategy for HIV and AIDS Prevention, Treatment and Care and Sexual and Reproductive Health and Rights among Key Populations'[4] which was approved by the SADC Ministers for Health and HIV and AIDS in 2017. This strategy focuses on policy, legal, institutional, and facility levels and aims to guide Member States in designing and implementing appropriate SRH and HIV prevention, treatment, and care programmes for key populations. We further discuss this strategy below.

While there is a relatively strong regional normative framework on SRHR in the African Union, the implementation of related resolutions and recommendations rests on the willingness of the individual states to lead on women's rights and to give priority to human rights at the country level. For example, despite most of the SADC member states having ratified the Maputo Protocol, which explicitly obliges state parties to create the legal, economic, and social conditions that enable women to exercise their sexual and reproductive rights with regard to family planning/contraception and safe abortion, there are currently only two SADC countries (Mozambique and South Africa) where abortion is permitted without restriction, within gestational limits, with the legal grounds for induced abortion varying considerably amongst the remainder of the countries in the region. While policy frameworks in SSA have paid attention to gender equality and SRHR, a gap has been noted in terms of focus on the most poor and vulnerable populations, resulting in inequitable access to SRHR services and information, as well as inadequate protection against catastrophic health spending for these populations in SSA (KIT Royal Tropical Institute, 2020).

## Who Are Key Populations?

The SADC Regional Strategy for Sexual and Reproductive Health and Rights (2019–2030) and the Regional Strategy for HIV and AIDS Prevention, Treatment, and Care and Sexual and Reproductive Health and Rights among Key Populations are valuable texts for understanding how the frameworks supporting policymakers understand or conceptualise vulnerability. In the latter document, "key populations" are narrowly defined as 'groups who, due to specific higher-risk behaviours, are at increased risk of HIV irrespective of the epidemic type or local context' (page 6). Sex workers are only considered such if they are 18 years and above. Children and adolescents under the age of 18 who exchange sex for money, goods, or favours are not included in the definition of sex workers since they are considered sexually exploited, as defined in the Convention on the Rights of the Child. However, in the same document, "young key populations" are understood as being 'individuals between the ages of 15 and 24 who, due to specific higher-risk behaviours, are at increased risk of HIV irrespective of the epidemic type or local context' but 'for the purposes of this strategy, key populations include (1) men who have sex with men, (2) people in prisons, (3) people who use drugs, (4) sex workers, and (5) transgender people'. We are keenly aware that young women under 18 years of age who engage in selling sex suffer sexual exploitation. However, the fact that they are also recognised as a young key population, as the above reflects, creates a definitional impasse which offers little guidance on the policy action required for AGYW who may fall outside of the box of a "sex worker" but who are involved in sexual-economic exchanges. These definitions have also meant that researchers have tended not to include adolescents (<18 years of age) who self-identify as being involved in selling sex (unless in the context of "transactional sex") in their studies due to the ethical complexities and, in some instances, mandatory reporting requirements, and this has led to an evidence-less vacuum in terms of what action is required to address these young women's extreme vulnerability. The strategy document goes on to define "vulnerable populations" as 'groups of people who are particularly vulnerable to HIV infection in certain situations or contexts, such as adolescents (particularly adolescent girls in sub-Saharan Africa), orphans, street children, people with disabilities, and migrant and mobile workers'. There is an added qualifier in the text which states that 'this strategy does not specifically address vulnerable populations, but it does note the specific vulnerabilities of young key populations', understanding vulnerability for YKPs to be linked to the 'legal and social issues related to their behaviours that increase their vulnerability to HIV' (page 6). In the context of the strategy document, key populations are primarily understood to be vulnerable to violence and to being made vulnerable through punitive and restrictive laws. We would argue, though, that this definition of "key populations", as well as being essentialising, does not really address what vulnerability is, who is made vulnerable, how they are rendered vulnerable, and why.

The widespread use of "key populations" as an approach for policy and programming related to SRHR can be seen both as a product and an element of reproduction of a narrow, biomedical, and behavioural risk-reduction-based approach to SRHR. Importantly, the "key populations" approach is part of the legacy of the HIV response, where those population groups who were most epidemiologically "at risk" of acquiring and transmitting the infection were defined. However, it has since been widely adopted across various institutional settings at both international and national levels and often guides the way various groups are targeted as being both "at risk" and "a risk" (as we explore further in Chapter 4). The key population approach is typical of a group-based approach to identify vulnerabilities, and as such, we argue, it misses the complexities involved in identifying how and why individuals get placed in positions of vulnerability to poor SRHR. In the second part of this chapter, we try and introduce a different approach to vulnerability to understand how this might better capture the ways in which certain people are placed in positions of vulnerability to negative SRHR outcomes.

## What Is Vulnerability?

The notion of vulnerability is itself open to debate both generally and within the context of health policies. And, as we have argued, SRHR is an area where the use of the concept of vulnerability has become ubiquitous, largely through the focus on HIV and AIDS and the definition of "key populations" or "vulnerable" groups within HIV and AIDS policies and programming and in the public health scholarship that frames the issue of HIV and AIDS. It can be argued, however, that certain uses of the notion of vulnerability are in fact counter-productive and may have unintended and sometimes negative consequences for health outcomes. These uses of vulnerability will not necessarily lead to increasing sexual and reproductive health rights, nor will they reach the most marginalised and those experiencing the most negative health outcomes.

An obvious difficulty with using any kind of vulnerability approach in health policy and programming is to understand who is vulnerable. And as Ruof (2004, p. 2) argues, 'difficulties in defining vulnerability have prompted discourse surrounding its utility as a qualifying factor in the allocation of health resources'. If health policies and allocation of resources are predicated upon this categorisation of vulnerability, then there is indeed an assumption that there will be measures in place to identify who is "vulnerable", and that vulnerability is something that can be identified in an individual (Luna, 2009). Thus, in our example of the key population approach to HIV and AIDS discussed above, there is the assumption that individuals can be easily identified as belonging to these key populations in order to be included in any programmes or resources targeted at them. This assumption, however, is problematic, 'relying as it does on a belief that vulnerability is a characteristic which is easily identifiable and objectifiable in an individual and neglect more complex relational and contextual causes and forms of vulnerability, simplifying and treating vulnerability as one dimensional rather than as a "layered concept"' (Freedman, 2019). Coming back again to the key populations approach, we can see the problematic nature of identifying vulnerability in this way: saying who is or who is not a sex worker, for example, in societies where there exists a whole continuum of sexual-economic exchanges (as we will discuss in Chapter 3).

One of the main tensions in the use of vulnerability is between seeing it as a characteristic of certain defined groups in society or understanding it as part of the universal human condition (Fineman, 2017) and an existential threat faced by all (Butler, 2015). In her work, Fineman talks about the ways in which all humans are vulnerable, but that this vulnerability is distributed differently according to social positions at various moments.

There is a tension between Fineman's approach, which calls for recognition of universal human vulnerability, and a seemingly contrary tendency in policy and practice to focus on the vulnerabilities of particular groups. Hence, we have seen an increase in the use of vulnerability as a concept aimed at differentiating between those who are deemed to be in need of support and those who are not. Within this approach, certain groups are frequently designated as more vulnerable when talking about focusing health care resources. According to Brown (2011, p. 313), 'the concept of vulnerability informs how we manage and classify people, justify state intervention in citizens' lives, allocate resources in society and define our social obligations'. These debates about who is more "vulnerable" and also the related question of who is more "deserving" of resources for health are particularly pointed where these resources are scarce, as in the case of many health systems in Southern Africa. This means that being identified as "vulnerable" is also highly politicised and may become a site of competition as various groups "compete" for the label in order to attract the funding and resources which are often directed to "vulnerable groups". This is particularly relevant in terms of donor funding and may also be seen in some cases to override or ignore national-level policymaking and funding allocation.

In many cases, this focus on "vulnerable groups" has been seen as a positive way of opening access to specific resources for people who are identified as belonging to these groups, for example, channelling more funding and support to sex workers, identified as a "key population" more vulnerable to infection by HIV. However, there are also criticisms of this group-led approach. One issue is that the process of "defining" a term or a group establishes limits and boundaries which tend to become fixed and static and often lead to a preoccupation with measurement rather than understanding, so that once a group has been named and its members identified, there is no possibility of understanding how and why individuals come to be in this group, nor how they move in and out of it at various junctures and moments in time. Returning once again to our example of sex workers as a key population, our research points to the complex social structures and individual stories which lead to women engaging in sexual-economic exchanges, as well as the ways in which they move in and out of different sexual relations and often maintain a principal non-transactional relationship as well as others for sexual economic exchange. In this scenario, identifying women as "sex workers" and placing them in a category of "vulnerable group" or "key population" acts to erase these complexities and represent and treat them in a unidimensional way. This, in turn, means that any policies or programmes aimed towards them cannot be fully adjusted or attuned to their real needs but are based on a "one size fits all" approach modelled on a non-existent "typical" sex worker, or they are left out entirely.

These fixed definitions of vulnerability and vulnerable groups also reinforce and reify existing gendered norms and representations. Feminist research points to the common association of vulnerability with femininity (and, by contrast, masculinity with dangerousness). Hollander (2001) notes that gendered understandings of vulnerability and dangerousness cannot be understood in isolation from other hierarchies of power and domination such as race, class, age etc. But often, the vulnerable groups' approach tends to simplify understandings and erase notions of intersectionality. Women might thus be classed as "vulnerable" to male violence without distinguishing how socio-economic differences, for example, render some women more likely to experience such violence than others and to have less recourse to support when they do.

The "vulnerable group" approach has thus been criticised for being linked to the stigmatisation, essentialisation, paternalistic targeting, and increased control and repression of those identified as vulnerable (Brown et al., 2017; Freedman, 2019; Reilly et al., 2022). Implicit in an understanding of vulnerability as pertaining (only) to particular groups is that vulnerability is a fixed property or, more specifically, a lack or deficiency of some groups and individuals compared to a presumed norm of "invulnerability". As Brown et al. (2017, p. 498) characterise the situation: 'while vulnerability has a deep discursive connection with connotations of empathy and compassion, and can be used in pursuit of enhanced support for certain individuals or groups, there is increasing attention to the ways in which it can also serve regulatory functions (…) when deployed in a normative way'. Viewed through a Foucauldian lens, the "production" of some groups as vulnerable is further implicated in the governance of populations and the extension of state bio-power (Butler, 2004). Labelling groups as vulnerable might thus be seen as a benevolent strategy in that it earmarks these groups for specific forms of support, but it can also be seen as a strategy of governmentality to better control the supposed "risks" that these groups pose. The labelling of vulnerable groups as "at risk" thus co-exists with representations of them as "a risk" to societies and social order. This relates to our discussion on the governance of HIV and AIDS (Chapter 4) and the way that the securitisation of HIV and AIDS led to certain groups being designated as "vulnerable" but also as a "risk" to society through their perceived likelihood of spreading disease. This in turn ties back to colonial tropes on certain groups, such as sex workers, as a risk to the health of society. 'The neoliberal focus upon "risk" marks a further turn in this biopolitical exercise and brings "vulnerability" – imagined threats to life – to the fore. Risk and vulnerability generate new forms through which both populations and individuals are governed through the mere potential (or alleged potential) for harm. Here, critical examination enables us to expose the ways that "vulnerability" works to oppress various groups' (Kaye et al., 2021, p. 72).

Kaye et al. (2021, p. 84) also point to the way in which it is impossible to fully escape the label of "vulnerable" once a person has been classified as such: 'vulnerability freezes identity, branding the person with their vulnerability and making it a permanent attribute of self, never moving it fully into the past tense'. They give the example of women living with HIV who are selected as peer "counsellors". These women are represented as being "empowered" by this new role, but they can only take up this role because they have been previously labelled as "vulnerable" and can never escape this prior labelling.

In contrast to "vulnerable group"-centred uses of the concept, a more radical definition of vulnerability takes as its point of departure the premise that vulnerability is a universal, inevitable, and constant human condition (Fineman, 2008; Mackenzie, 2014; Turner, 2006) Rejecting 'the impoverished legal subject of Locke and liberal thought with its characteristics of autonomy and independence' Fineman (2013, p. 31) calls on critical legal scholars to argue for an alternative conception of the legal subject that is 'flexible, powerful, and able to incorporate a panoply of circumstances and positions'. In doing so, she draws on feminist theorisations of care and dependency (Fineman, 2004; Kittay, 2020 [1999]; Tronto, 1993; 2013), as well as feminist economics and other critical perspectives that reject the assumption of the self-interested, rationally calculating "economic man" as the defining feature of human behaviour and source of the contractual view of society and social relations (Ferber & Nelson, 2020; Fineman & Dougherty, 2005; Folbre 2001; Wærness, 1984).

In Fineman's conceptualisation, 'the human condition is one of *universal* and *continuous* vulnerability' (Fineman, 2017, p. 134, emphasis added). It 'carries with it the imminent or ever- present possibility of harm, injury, or misfortune' (Fineman, 2010, p. 30) through external and internal forces, including the passing of time and eventually death. In this respect, Fineman's assumption of universal vulnerability resembles arguments made by Judith Butler regarding precarious life (2004). However, while vulnerability is universal and constant, Fineman argues, it is also experienced differently, depending on the particularities of individual embodiment and positions 'within webs of economic and institutional relationships' and 'the quality and quantity of resources we possess or can command' (Fineman, 2010, p. 30).

While all human beings stand in a position of constant vulnerability, we are individually positioned differently. We have different forms of embodiment and are also differently situated within webs of economic and institutional relationships. As a result, our vulnerabilities range in magnitude and potential at the individual level. Vulnerability, therefore, is both universal and particular; it is experienced uniquely by each of us. Important in regard to this particular point is the fact that our individual experience of vulnerability varies according to the quality and quantity of resources we possess or can command. While society cannot eradicate our vulnerability, it can and does mediate, compensate, and lessen our vulnerability through programmes, institutions, and structures. (Fineman, 2010, p. 269). This understanding of vulnerability is, we argue, useful for moving beyond a "group"-based approach and understanding individual positioning and the ways that people are made vulnerable through intersecting structures of inequality and discrimination. This is particularly relevant, as we discuss through the book, for understandings of vulnerability to poor SRH outcomes.

Although society cannot eradicate vulnerability, it can and does mediate, compensate, and lessen the consequences of vulnerability. Importantly, the counterpoint to vulnerability is not invulnerability but resilience. As Fineman describes it, 'resilience … provides an individual with the means and ability to recover from harm, setbacks and the misfortunes that affect our lives' (2017, p. 149). Resilience is acquired over time within social structures and institutions (family, market, or state); it depends on the quantity and quality of the resources we have access to and shapes our capacity to take advantage of opportunities and cope with adversity. It follows that unequal access to societal structures or unequal allocations of privilege and power within social structures diminishes resilience (2017, p. 147).

Resilience has also become a commonplace term and goal within a neo-liberal framework, as we discuss further below, where individual resilience to various types of shocks is praised. But in contrast to this neo-liberal view, Fineman (2017) argues that the focus on individual resilience can obscure the larger structural inequalities and systemic injustices that shape people's lives. In other words, individuals cannot develop resilience without the necessary resources to do so, and this depends on reallocation by the state to ensure that everyone has equal access to such resources.

## Situated Intersectionality

One of the criticisms of Fineman's idea of universal human vulnerability is that this conception has the potential to erase key differences between individuals and tend towards an unwarranted universalism. As an antidote to this somewhat justified criticism, we can turn to intersectional analyses and see how an intersectionality lens can be applied to feminist vulnerability theory. Intersectionality, as first proposed by Crenshaw (1989), aims to analyse and understand the ways in which different structures of social inequality, discrimination, and oppression overlap and interact in multiple and complex ways in "interlocking systems of oppression" (Hill Collins, 1993, p. 615). As Symington (2004, p. 5) points out, 'the rich descriptions produced through intersectional analysis illuminate the actors, institutions, policies and norms that intertwine to create a given situation. Such textured analyses are critical to our ability to effect progressive change in the face of the fundamentalist forces, neoliberal economic policies, militarization, new technologies, entrenched patriarchy and colonialism, and new imperialism that threaten women's rights and sustainable development today'.

Intersectionality encompasses a range of theoretical and conceptual tools (Lutz et al., 2011; Anthias, 2013) and can be interpreted in a variety of ways. Perhaps most useful for understanding and situating vulnerability is the concept of situated intersectionality developed by Yuval-Davis (2015). This idea of situated intersectionality, which emphasises the contextual and situated nature of the social categorisations that exist and of the systems of inequalities and oppressions within which individuals are situated, allows us also to employ an intersectional analysis in the countries of Southern Africa with which we are concerned here without falling into the trap of merely "importing" Eurocentric or colonialist forms of analysis. As Meer and Müller (2017, p. 3) argue, 'the range of social categories that inform individuals' lived experiences and the production of social relations on the African continent may be considerably different to the staples of race, class and gender in the existing, mostly American-and European-focused literature'. This consideration is highly relevant here, and as our research shows, certain categorisations which have been frequently under-analysed or absent in Eurocentric intersectional analyses may be much more important in our settings. Age, for example, has emerged in much of our research as a key axis of inequality and domination (as we discuss concerning relations between older and younger women who sell sex in Chapter 3), a reflection also raised by other African feminist scholars (Prah, 2017).

Situated intersectionality allows us to understand the mutual constitution of social divisions and hierarchies, which as Yuval-Davis (2015, p. 94) explains, 'the particular nuanced and contested meanings of particular social locations in particular historical moments, within particular social, economic and political contexts in which some social divisions have more saliency and effect'. She explains that situated intersectionality must take translocality seriously, that is, the way particular social categories and divisions have different meanings and different relations of power in different spaces. It must also consider seriously how these meanings and relations of power change with scale (translocality) and over time (transtemporality).

A situated intersectional analysis calls for an examination of the operation of complex systems of intersecting dominations within a specific local, national, and regional context shaped by, for example, the legacy of apartheid or colonial domination (and ongoing neo-colonial forms of oppression). As Walker et al. (2017, p. 93) argue in their analysis of the vulnerabilities of migrant women selling sex in South Africa, while acknowledging all the debates around intersectionality, this lens is useful in that it allows us 'to understand experience and meaning within specific social contexts (in this case, those associated with peripheral urban lives) and though a lens or lenses that bring together theoretical concepts with shifting embodied practices'. A situated intersectionality lens is clearly useful in understanding how and why refugee women are placed in positions of vulnerability to sexual and gender-based violence, as we discuss in Chapter 5 of this book.

There have been calls for vulnerability theory to take account of identity power relations (Cooper, 2015), for vulnerability analysis to focus on "vulnerable life situations" (Virokannas et al., 2020), and, if formulating targeted protections, to address particular threats (Kohn, 2014). These, we argue, signpost the route to reconciling vulnerability and intersectionality theory in ways that eschew counterproductive identity politics and essentialist logic (Reilly et al., 2022).

Ultimately, they are an argument for making context-specific vulnerability analysis the most important part of vulnerability theory. We thus bring this analytical lens to the remainder of the chapters in our book.

## Resilience and Essential Conditions for the Achievement of Sexual and Reproductive Rights

> By now it should be clear that resilience is not a thing, nor is there "one" logic of resilience that informs all instances of its usage.
>
> (Humbert & Joseph, 2019, p. 215)

We talked above about the opposite of vulnerability in Fineman's understanding, which is the concept of resilience. But like definitions and understandings of vulnerability, the concept of resilience is also broad and open to many different interpretations. One of the main critiques of the idea of resilience has been that it is used in a neo-liberal way to encourage individual action and to shift the responsibility for achieving more positive life or health outcomes onto individuals. We have argued that, in fact, Fineman's insistence on the role of states and governments in redistributing resources in order for all to have the necessary resources for resilience links this idea back to that of social structures and collective responsibility. But it is important to underline this point and to emphasise that when we talk about SRHR resilience, we are making an argument not about individuals taking responsibility for their own SRHR but about the need to challenge existing structures of inequality and to hold states and governments responsible for putting in place policies to do so.

This critique of neo-liberal conceptions of resilience links to another criticism of Fineman's vulnerability theory, which concerns the lack of scope for collective agency and engagement with the political, which are serious limitations of vulnerability theory, which tends to deal with individuals and groups in their relations with institutions/states as objects of policy intervention rather than as political and civic subjects. This raises the question: who shall hold the state to account and push it to become more responsive in non-oppressive ways? If we look at the development and history of human rights, this "push" has depended on the mobilisation and collective agency of civil society, in particular women's and anti-racist movements, among others (Reilly, 2009; Weldon & Htun, 2013). In this regard, Turner (2006, p. 32) provides a valuable amendment to vulnerability theory, firstly by reaffirming the indispensable role of civil liberties in facilitating individual and collective action to hold the state to account; and secondly, by recognising – as part of a necessary political-sociological process – collective agency and engagement to continually 'repair and redesign' precarious state, institutional, and policy responses to human vulnerability. This is again important in our research settings where collective action by women's movements, for example, has brought about important institutional changes which might in some ways contribute to reducing women's vulnerability and increasing resistance – for example, by campaigning for legal and political reform on access to safe abortion or mobilising to highlight the issue of sexual and gender-based violence and call for action to prevent it.

Fineman's vulnerability analysis, deployed through a lens of situated intersectionality that reveals inequality, injustice, and harm as the result of institutional arrangements, is especially useful in analysing the relation between the individual, state, and society. Moreover, it shifts the responsibility and the blame from the victim to the institutions that partly produce or facilitate the conditions that give rise to harms while also failing to respond adequately to them. The state must then be involved, not only to grant rights but also to support individuals in claiming these rights. Using situated intersectionality to think about not only situations of vulnerability but also the transformation of these, including institutional transformation (Moore & Himonga, 2017), can be seen as a productive way forward to analyse vulnerability in a context-specific way. This approach can understand individual and institutional arrangements in specific contexts and can encompass both individual autonomy and agency, as well as the importance of social movements to work towards reducing vulnerability and improving resilience. In the following chapters, we explore different SRHR issues through this lens in order to try and point out better ways to address these challenges.

## Conclusion

In this chapter, we have tried to describe the ways in which the existing policy frameworks for SRHR can be criticised for adopting a group-based approach to the identification of "vulnerable groups" and how this has been shaped by donors and multilateral organisations (as we discuss further in Chapter 4). This approach, we have argued, tends to essentialise vulnerability as a characteristic of pre-defined groups and thus leaves no room for a real understanding of how people move in and out of vulnerable situations depending on a range of social categorisations and inequalities. It also reinforces a tendency to ignore the complexities of individual situations and to gloss over any instances where there are clear binaries or divisions between groups, which leads to definitional impasses offering little guidance on the policy action required. We argue instead for an approach to vulnerability based on a situated intersectionality framework, showing how a range of intersecting axes of inequality will place individuals in situations of vulnerability and how this will vary across geographical and temporal locations. This approach, we argue, is more productive in understanding how some people experience negative SRHR outcomes and in attempting to design policies which will address these.

## Notes

1 As of the end of 2023, Madagascar has signed but not ratified, Malawi has ratified but not signed and Botswana has neither signed nor ratified.
2 Critiques of the way in which gender has been integrated into development policy (and other policy areas) have pointed to the way in which "mainstreaming" has become a "buzzword" (Cornwall, 2007) which is used indiscriminately across policy documents, and which has, in many cases, lost any real meaning.
3 https://www.sadc.int/document/strategy-sexual-and-reproductive-health-and-rights-sadc-region-2019-2030
4 https://www.2gether4srhr.org/resources/regional-strategy-for-hiv-prevention-treatment-and-care-and-sexual-and-reproductive-health-and-rights-among-key-populations

## References

Anthias, F. (2013). Intersectional what? Social divisions, intersectionality and levels of analysis. *Ethnicities*, *13*(1), 3–19.

Brown, K. (2011). 'Vulnerability': Handle with care. *Ethics and Social Welfare*, *5*(3), 313–321.

Brown, K., Ecclestone, K., & Emmel, N. (2017). The many faces of Vulnerability. *Social Policy and Society*, *16*(3), 497–510.

Butler, J. (2004). *Precarious life: The powers of mourning and violence*. Verso.

Butler, J. (2015). Performative agency. In *The limits of performativity* (pp. 10–24). Routledge.

Cooper, F. R. (2015). Always already suspect: Revising vulnerability theory. *North Carolina Law Review*, *93(5)*, 1339–1380.

Cornwall, A. (2007). Buzzwords and fuzzwords: Deconstructing development discourse. *Development in Practice*, *17*(4-5), 471–484.

Crenshaw, K. (1989). Demarginalising the intersection of race and sex: A black feminist critique of antidiscrimination, feminist theory and antiracist politics. University of Chicago Legal Forum, 1989(1), 139–167.

Ferber, M. A., & Nelson, J. A. (Eds.). (2020). *Feminist economics today: Beyond economic man*. University of Chicago Press.

Fineman, M. A. (2004). *The autonomy myth: A theory of dependency*. The New Press.

Fineman, M. A. (2008). The vulnerable subject: Anchoring equality in the human condition. *Yale Journal of Law and Feminism*, *20*(1), 1–23.

Fineman, M. A. (2010). The vulnerable subject and the responsive state. *Emory Law Journal*, *60*(2), 251–275. Emory Public Law Research Paper No. 10-130. Available at SSRN: https://ssrn.com/abstract=1694740.

Fineman, M. A. (2013). Feminist theory in law: The difference it makes. In *Feminist legal theories* (pp. 213–235). Routledge.

Fineman, M. (2017). Vulnerability and inevitable inequality. *Oslo Law Review*, *4*(3), 133–149.

Fineman, M. A., & Dougherty, T. (Eds.). (2005). *Feminism confronts homo economicus: Gender, law, and society*. Cornell University Press.

Folbre, N. (2001). *The invisible heart: Economics and family values*. The New Press.

Freedman, J. (2019). The uses and abuses of "Vulnerability" in EU asylum and refguee protection: Protecting women or reducing autonomy? *Papeles Del CEIC*, *2019*(1), 1–15.

Hill Collins, P. (1993). Black feminist thought in the matrix of domination. In C. C. Lemert (Ed.), *Social theory: The multicultural and classic readings* (pp. 615–625). Westview Press.

Hollander, J. A. (2001). Vulnerability and dangerousness: The construction of gender through conversation about violence. *Gender & Society*, *15*(1), 83–109.

Humbert, & Joseph (2019). Introduction: The politics of resilience: Problematising current approaches. *Resilience*, *7*(3), 215–223.

Kaye, K., Amuchástegui, A., George, A., & Navarro, T. (2021). Neoliberal vulnerability and the vulnerability of neoliberalism. In E. Bernstein, & J. R. Jakobsen (Eds.), *Paradoxes of neoliberalism: Sex, gender and possibilities for justice* (pp. 71–108). Routledge.

KIT Royal Tropical Institute. (2020). Final Report: Regional Context Analysis of SRHR in Sub-Saharan Africa. Amsterdam, https://www.kit.nl/wp-content/uploads/2022/02/Final-report_SRHR-context-analysis-SSA.pdf

Kittay, N. A. (2020). [1999]. *Love's labor: Essays on women, equality and dependency*. Routledge.

Kohn, N. A. (2014). Vulnerability theory and the role of Government. *Yale Journal of Law and Feminism*, *26*(1), 1–27.

Luna, F. (2009). Elucidating the concept of vulnerability: Layers not labels. *International Journal of Feminist Approaches to Bioethics*, *2*(1), 121–139. http://www.jstor.org/stable/40339200

Mackenzie, C. (2014). The importance of relational autonomy and capabilities for an ethics of vulnerability. In C. Mackenzie, W. Rogers, & S. Dodds (Eds.), *Vulnerability: New essays in ethics and feminist philosophy* (pp. 33–59). Oxford University Press.

Meer, T., & Müller, A. (2017). Considering intersectionality in Africa. *Agenda*, *31*(1), 3–4.

Moore, E., & Himonga, C. (2017). Centring the intersection of race, class, and gender when a customary marriage ends. *Agenda*, *31*(1), 104–115. https://doi.org/10.1080/10130950.2017.1357375.

Prah, E. (2017). Stratifications of blackness: Meditations on the intersect of gender, race and age. *Agenda*, *31*(1), 71–77. https://doi.org/10.1080/10130950.2017.1354441.

Reilly, N. (2009). *Women's human rights: Seeking gender justice in a globalizing age*. Polity Press.

Reilly, N., Bjørnholt, M., & Tastsoglou, E. (2022). Vulnerability, precarity and intersectionality: A critical review of three key concepts for understanding gender-based violence in migration contexts. In J. Freedman, N. Sahraoui & E. Tastsoglou (Eds.), *Gender-based violence in migration: Interdisciplinary, feminist and intersectional approaches* (pp. 29–56). Palgrave Macmillan. https://doi.org/10.1007/978-3-031-07929-0_2

Ruof, M. C. (2004). Vulnerability, vulnerable populations, and policy. *Kennedy Institute of Ethics Journal*, *14*(4), 411–425.

Symington, A. (2004). *Intersectionality: A tool for gender and economic justice*. Association for Women in Development.

Tronto, J. C. (1993). *Moral boundaries: A political argument for an ethic of care*. Psychology Press.

Tronto, J. C. (2013). *Caring democracy: Markets, equality, and justice*. NYU Press.

Turner, B.S. (2006). *Vulnerability and human rights*. Penn State University Press.

Virokannas, E., Liuski, S., & Kuronen, M. (2020). The contested concept of vulnerability – A literature review. *European Journal of Social Work*, *23*(2), 327–339. https://doi.org/10.1080/13691457.2018.1508001.

Wærness, K. (1984). The rationality of caring. *Economic and Industrial Democracy*, *5*(2), 185–211.

Walker, R., Vearey, J., & Nencel, L. (2017). Negotiating the city: Exploring the intersecting vulnerabilities of non-national migrant mothers who sell sex in Johannesburg, South Africa. *Agenda, 31*(1), 91–103. https://doi.org/10.1080/10130950.2017.1338858.

Weldon, S. L., & Htun, M. (2013). Feminist mobilisation and progressive policy change: Why governments take action to combat violence against women. *Gender and Development, 21*(2), 231–247. http://www.jstor.org/stable/24697245

Yuval-Davis, N. (2015). Situated intersectionality and social inequality. *Raisons Politiques*, 58, 91–100.

# 3

# VULNERABILITY ACROSS THE SEXUAL-ECONOMIC EXCHANGE CONTINUUM

## Introduction

The legacy of colonialism on a continent worst affected by the AIDS pandemic has profoundly shaped contemporary societal attitudes towards women engaged in sexual exchanges for money, goods, and other forms of payment or services in sub-Saharan Africa (Aantjes et al., 2022a). Young women involved in these sexual exchanges have been the focus of numerous programmes, policies, and funding initiatives which have been defined and put in place explicitly in response to their heightened vulnerability to acquiring HIV (Dellar et al., 2015). As these programmes have developed, a clear distinction between "commercial sex work" and "transactional sex" has been established based on the argument that these types of sexual exchanges are conceptually and practically distinct and have different consequences for women's health and well-being, with the two groups targeted by different public health interventions and approaches (Crankshaw & Freedman, 2023). Within these conceptual regimes, "sex work" is considered to be a formalised and commercial negotiation of sex in return for payment, whereas "transactional" sex is understood as informal and explicitly non-commercial, where love and trust may sometimes be present. With respect to transactional sex, economic support is understood within the context of an intimate relationship, while sex work is viewed as an explicit purchase of sex, and it is implied that these exchanges occur outside the bounds of an intimate relationship. In this chapter, we will question the value of this distinction in advancing our understanding of vulnerability and informing our responses to poor SRH. In doing so, we will examine the continuum[1] of sexual-economic exchanges that exist and the ways in which women involved may be placed in

DOI: 10.4324/9781003414698-3

situations of vulnerability. We will argue that a group-based approach (being categorised as a "sex worker" – or not) defined by HIV risk and health indicators does not provide a comprehensive understanding of the ways in which intersectional inequalities constrain women's choices in engaging in sexual-economic exchange or not and the ways in which this impacts their full range of SRHR. Broadening the focus beyond HIV and health risk frees us to examine the intersections of the full range of structures and conditions that, combined, underpin differences in vulnerability and inequalities in health and well-being.

## Transactional Sex Versus Sex Work

Social science and feminist scholarship has long engaged with the fluidity of transactional sexual relationships within a diverse array of situations and has examined the gendered structures of power within which these relationships are established (Formson & Hillhorst, 2016; McMillan et al., 2018; Tabet, 2005, 2012). Strong arguments, however, persist, particularly in public health scholarship focusing on sub-Saharan Africa and within various public health programmes (and particularly those originating in an HIV-focused agenda) against conflating transactional sex with sex work (UNAIDS 2018). Several pragmatic and positive intentions behind this mobilisation of a category of transactional sex as distinct from sex work can be acknowledged. It offers a way to escape Western misrepresentation of the complexities of sexual relations in African societies (Ankomah, 1999) and to avoid stigmatising women who do not self-identify as sex workers but who are engaged in informal sexual exchange relationships. It also circumvents the labels of "sex worker" or "prostitute" while still ensuring inclusion of a spectrum of women involved in sexual economic exchanges in datasets examining risk. Others have argued that the conceptual separation of transactional sex from commercial sex work works to 'bestow cultural legitimacy on some locally specific forms of paid sex' (McMillan et al., 2018, p. 1517) and to position these as part of local cultures rather than within economic structures. However, we argue that it is equally important not to reify local cultures and the forms of sexual-economic exchange which might occur within them but to seek to understand how local cultures and economies interact with wider global economic structures as determinants of sexual-economic exchange (Freedman et al., 2021). Our ongoing research with women engaged in the continuum of sexual-economic exchange in several Southern African countries has led us to question the utility of these distinctions in practice (Crankshaw et al., 2021; Crankshaw & Freedman, 2023; Freedman et al., 2020a, 2021), with resultant programmes defined for and aimed at either "sex workers" or women engaged in "transactional sex".

The research started from a point where, focusing on "key populations" as mentioned earlier in the book, we drew on the already defined categories of sex workers and women engaging in transactional sex to identify and try to understand the experiences of our participants. But we quickly realised, firstly, that there was a huge diversity of experience within the group identified as "sex workers", and secondly, multiple similarities and shared experiences between those who were identified/self-identified as sex workers and those who were not. This led us to question the value of adopting a group-based approach (or quantification of the idea of vulnerability) based on identification or non-identification as a commercial sex worker. And indeed, who confers this categorisation? Must a woman actively identify as a sex worker to be considered, or are women classed in groups based on their behavioural characteristics? Irrespective, this group-based approach, which has echoes in the control of infectious diseases in the colonial past and which has been inherited from HIV interventions, does not, we argue, take into account the complexities of reasons for engaging in sexual-economic exchange and the impacts of this on women's SRHR. The similar vulnerabilities experienced by all of the women we interviewed are determined not by how they identify or are identified, or by their belonging to one of these pre-defined categories, but by intersectional axes of inequality and domination such as social class, ethnicity, migration/citizenship status and, in particular, age. Understanding their situation within these axes, which cut across all forms of sexual-economic exchange, would, we believe, be more productive in designing policies and programmes to reduce vulnerabilities and increase resilience in order to improve SRHR more comprehensively. Analyses such as these work to strengthen the response to the broader social determinants underlying the SRHR agenda.

While we recognise the utility of the categories of "transactional sex" as distinct from "commercial sex work" in the early days when the HIV pandemic was experienced as an unprecedented crisis in a rapidly evolving global health environment, we argue these may no longer be the most helpful way of informing a more comprehensive SRH response (including HIV) to reduce vulnerability and strengthen women's resilience. We thus argue in this chapter that we need to move beyond a purely epidemiological or "health"-based focus which considers sex work/transactional sex as "risks" for women's and girls' health, to focus more broadly on the sexual and reproductive health and rights of those involved, and to propose policy and programmatic entry points for addressing situated vulnerabilities. Emphasising the importance of rights and the need for an intersectional approach to the realisation of these rights allows us to now more closely interrogate these conceptual boundaries within the broader SRHR context. These considerations are vitally important with growing levels of poverty and fragmented family structures in many countries and increasingly youthful participation in sexual-economic exchanges. These contexts require us to critically examine the value of adhering to group-based categorisations in understanding the SRH vulnerabilities of young women participating in these exchanges. This debate is particularly important in the context of very young women, where gendered inequalities and young age interact to create particular situations of vulnerability for poor SRHR.

Employing feminist interpretations of vulnerability theory (Fineman, 2017), as discussed in Chapter 2, we can conclude that a shift in dialogue from understanding vulnerabilities as based on identities or categories and towards a situated intersectional understanding (Yuval-Davis, 2015) of how and why individuals become situated in vulnerable positions would allow us to better understand the impacts of various axes of inequality, such as age, class, ethnicity, or citizenship/migration status, on the ways that women engaging in sexual-economic exchange become vulnerable to negative SRH outcomes, including sexual and gender-based violence (SGBV).

## The Framing of the Debate: Post-colonialism and Medicalisation

There is a well-established international social science and public health literature focusing on formal/commercial sex work, as well as literature related to "transactional sex" in its broader sense (Cole, 2004, 2009; Hunter, 2002; Manganja, 2007; Schoepf, 1988, 2009; White & Kamye, 2022), including 'both affective and commercially motivated sexual relations, as well as sex within non-exclusive, exclusive, and concurrent relationships' (McMillan et al., 2018, p. 1522). In HIV-related research based in SSA, however, transactional sex, defined as 'a sexual relationship or act(s), outside of marriage or sex work, motivated primarily by the expectation of material gain, where love and trust are also sometimes present (involved/concerned/at play)' (Stoebenau et al., 2016, p. 193) and "commercial" sex work, or 'any agreement between two or more persons in which the objective is exclusively limited to the sexual act and ends with that and which involves preliminary negotiations for a price'[2] (UNAIDS, 2000, p. 13), tend to be presented as conceptually distinct practices. This categorisation leads to women engaging in sexual-economic exchange being assigned, in programmes and policies (and law), to one or other of the categories and thus treated differently and with varied benefits and disadvantages.

Those categorised as sex workers have been found to have a higher prevalence of HIV compared to people in the general population, and are therefore understood to have a heightened risk of HIV, and so a case is made to track these groups for epidemiological purposes. However, in sub-Saharan Africa, the fact that women (and especially young women) are still the population group most likely to acquire HIV (UNAIDS, 2022) has led to many research projects and interventions focusing on women's supposedly "risky" sexual behaviours (Anderson, 2015), which make them vulnerable to HIV infection. This, in turn, has structured a group-based approach which understands risk in terms of belonging to a pre-identified group of "sex workers" or women engaging in transactional sex. In fact, a 2018 UNAIDS report on transactional sex and HIV risk underlined the need to better measure and categorise transactional sex so as to ensure 'transactional sex is distinguished from sex work' (UNAIDS, 2018, p. 16). However, as argued above, both the differences within and the similarities between these two categories render the distinction so blurred that it can no longer be seen as useful.

We appreciate that these distinctions sought to situate and understand different forms of sexual-economic exchange within a particular context where HIV was seen as the main SRHR challenge. Further, this HIV-related research and programming is located within a region where there are various levels of domestic, regional, and international political regimes which present varying hostilities or resistance to sex work. And importantly, this is a region where colonialities of power, knowledge, and subjectivity are ever present (Ndlovu-Gatsheni, 2013) and impact heavily on the dominant framings of sexuality and sexual and gender relations, including the framings of sex work. At the domestic level, the legal systems of the majority of countries in sub-Saharan Africa reflect their colonial legacies, in which "prostitution" is explicitly criminalised or living off the proceeds of selling sex made illegal. Often, this legislation is rather vague in its definitions of prostitution, employs colonial language of "immorality", and links sex work to out-of-marriage sexual relationships (Aantjes et al., 2022a). In Zimbabwe, for example, the legislation relating to sex work explicitly defines engagement in "extra-marital sex" for money or reward as the conduct of a "prostitute" (Criminal Codification and Reform Act [Chapter 9, p. 23]).[3]

In many countries in sub-Saharan Africa, sex work is stigmatised and is viewed as a Western import and "unAfrican" (Mgbako & Smith, 2009). In some cases, the rejection and stigmatisation of sex workers has been reinforced at the highest level of government, with at least two African presidents publicly proclaiming the threat of "prostitution" to the moral order and cultural fabric of society (Mgbako & Smith, 2009); sex workers are described as "unhealthy women" responsible for the spread of disease (Mgbako, 2019). On an international level, it can be argued that these colonialist views, which criminalised and stigmatised sex work, have been reproduced through HIV and AIDS interventions (Flint & Hewitt, 2015). For example, the early 2000s saw the rollout of the US President's Emergency Plan for AIDS Relief (PEPFAR) programme, which emerged as a major funder of a region with insufficient domestic resources to respond to the unfolding health crisis. However, as part of the then US Administration's conditions for the rollout of funds for HIV care and ARV treatment, grant recipients were explicitly forbidden from allowing sex workers to be enrolled in care (Ditmore & Allman, 2013). If grant recipients did not comply, they risked having their funding entirely withdrawn.

This type of positioning echoes colonial tropes on African sexuality and positions those such as sex workers who engaged in "risky" sex as morally at fault for the spread of the infection (Flint & Hewitt, 2015) and whose "behaviour" needs to be curbed. As Merten and Haller (2007) argue, the messages about "risk behaviour" central to HIV prevention programmes lead to the internationalisation of these messages as moral norms, which may also contribute to the unwillingness of many women involved in sexual economic exchange to self-identify or to be identified as sex workers. Rejection or invisibilisation of sex work can also be noted in some African research, notably that of African feminists and gender researchers (Richter, 2012), who reject sex work as a colonial import/construct (Hill, 2020) and oppose the importation of European feminist paradigms (Akin-Aina, 2011), such as that of pro-sex work feminists. This means that, as Mgbako argues, 'African feminist scholars, with a few notable exceptions, have largely remained silent on the issue of sex work' (Mgbako, 2016, p. 11). This silence has left a void which, in the context of the HIV and AIDS pandemic, was quickly filled by international public health scholarship and interventions which treat sex work in terms of "risk", focusing on the "sex" and not the structural conditions of this work and the discrimination and inequality which these might engender (Mgbako, 2016). It is also in this context that the division between commercial sex work and transactional sex has been established and continues to be reproduced and reinforced through programmes based on groups identified as being "at risk".

It is also in this context that the concept of transactional sex has been defined within the biomedical and public health research on HIV in sub-Saharan Africa, in opposition to the term of sex work (UNAIDS 2018). In making distinctions around the non-commercial aspect of transactional sex and the ways in which transactional sexual relationships involve emotional and not only economic dimensions, the proponents of this conceptual distinction argue that they have sought to avoid misrepresenting or stigmatising those women involved in such exchanges as "sex workers" (McMillan et al., 2018). But perhaps we can argue that paradoxically, in doing so, they reinforce the stigmatising category of sex work and create a monolithic categorisation which both elides the differences between sex workers and narrows the space for more productive discussion around sex workers' rights. In contexts where sex work is (partially) criminalized, as in most of sub-Saharan Africa, the fact of separating transactional sex from sex work might act to polarise the debates over criminalisation by making sex work distinct from other forms of sexual-economic exchange which occur widely in society. It is important to note that the discourses around the heightened "risks" encountered by sex workers occur in this context of criminalisation, and it is interesting to consider whether this distinction would have been established or maintained if sex work was decriminalised. This might suggest that rather than continue to uphold the categorisation and identification of sex work, it would be more productive to work collectively to de-criminalise all forms of sexual-economic exchange as part of a larger programme of supporting resilience and rights.

## Situated Vulnerabilities for Women Engaged in Sexual-Economic Exchange

As we have discussed, arguments have been made against conflating the two categories of sex work and transactional sex since this 'confounds efforts to track and understand the role that transactional sexual relationships may play in HIV risk, and stymies effective intervention efforts' (Stoebenau et al., 2016, p. 187). Here, the distinction is grounded in differences relating to self-identification (or not) as a sex worker: Exchanges of goods or money linked explicitly to sex versus exchanges of goods or money implicit in a relationship including sex; and little shared emotional intimacy versus some shared emotional intimacy (UNAIDS, 2018). In considering these criteria for distinction in our research, we question their applicability or usefulness in understanding and addressing vulnerabilities. Whilst the young women we interviewed across various countries were variously self-identified or not self-identified as sex workers, their experiences of sexual-economic exchanges were overlapping and often indistinguishable. We thus cite here women who do or do not identify themselves as sex workers to show the commonalities of their experiences and to make a case that it is more productive to consider the continuum of sexual-economic exchange.

Factors which had more impact on women's experiences than self-identification or not were their position in terms of social class and economic resources, age, family relationships, and migration status, with the youngest and poorest women and those with no legal citizenship status being most vulnerable to SGBV, for example (Crankshaw et al., 2021; Freedman et al., 2021). Moreover, the structuring effect of policy and programmatic interventions based on the sex work/transactional sex binary acted both to create and reinforce various forms of vulnerability. In this section, we use a situated intersectional analysis to apply to our data from Madagascar, Mozambique, Zambia, and Zimbabwe to understand how and why young women become involved in sexual-economic exchange and what this means for them. In one of the following sections, we will look more closely at sexual-economic exchanges for women with precarious legal status, as is the case of young woman refugees in South Africa.

Adopting a situated intersectional analysis allows us to understand why young women become involved in sexual-economic exchange and how they become and remain vulnerable in these situations. Across all of our studies, we found that economic insecurities were a major reason for engaging in these sexual relationships. Many young women told us that they engage in sexual-economic exchange in order to be able to buy basic necessities for themselves or their families or to fund their schooling. As one young woman in Madagascar explained:

> We don't do it because we want to! We need money because our parents can't provide for us, so we have no other choice. And sometimes when girls get pregnant they have to look after their own children because the father of the child won't do it. So then they need the money even more.

A 17-year-old woman in Zimbabwe told us: 'We didn't have money for school fees so I just thought it was better to be a sex worker, for me to be able to fend for myself'.

The fact that sexual-economic exchange is a well-known means of supporting girls' education was widely acknowledged in our studies. School girls interviewed in Antsiranana, Madagascar, explained that men knew what time school finished and waited outside the school gates for the students to come out. 'They hoot their horns and they manage to find girls who need money' (16-year-old woman, Madagascar).

Economic insecurity underpins participation in sexual-economic exchanges and a lack of formal employment opportunities, particularly for young women. The types of mainly informal employment in which many women are engaged do not provide sufficient income for basic necessities. In fact, many of the young women we interviewed participated in different forms of informal employment, such as street vending and hair styling, or engaged in local agricultural work, but did not make sufficient money from these activities and so used sexual-economic exchange as a means to top up their income as economic need arose. They might engage in these types of relationships even when they were also doing other forms of work, because these alone were not sufficient for economic survival. In Zimbabwe, young women who self-identified as "sex workers" or as explicitly selling sex also frequently reported other concurrent forms of income including cooking, trading, street vending, and hair braiding, for example. We also found a fluidity of engagement in sexual-economic exchanges across all country contexts, which could both be part of longer term sexual relationships or once-off encounters, with young women moving in and out of the different types of sexual relationships, sometimes concurrently.

Women's involvement in sexual-economic exchange may be reinforced by a gendered segregation of employment, which means that although unemployment is high among all young people, economic opportunities are even more limited for young women. This gendered segregation of labour is linked to norms concerning women's and men's physical capabilities and the suitability of certain jobs. As one young man in Madagascar explained to us:

> It's girls who are much more involved with it (sexual-economic exchange) because boys find work much more easily as they have much more physical strength.
>
> *(22-year-old man, Madagascar)*

Sexual-economic exchange is also rooted in unequal gender norms, which prescribe particular roles for women and men within sexual relationships. Early marriage and pressure to demonstrate fertility to fulfil their roles as women within their society are common in all the country contexts. The positive value attributed to heterosexual relations within these traditional gender norms may push young women into early sexual relationships within which they have little power or choice. Our research in Madagascar suggests that young women have their first sexual relationship at around 13 or 14 years old, although it is not that rare for girls to start having sex at the age of ten. In Zimbabwe, sexual debut typically occurred between 12 and 15 years, and in our Zambian research, sexual debut was as early as 11 years; sometimes sexual debut was reported to have occurred in the context of sexual-economic exchange. Generally, participants reported a few years between sexual debut (which often coincided with early marriage) and selling sex, citing economic reasons – primarily the financial responsibilities attached to motherhood – for starting to sell sex and reinforcing our argument for a focus on the full continuum of sexual-economic exchange.

> Mostly I just lack money and that is why we go for these men on the streets who can give you something for quick sex. If I was to find another source of income or a man to marry me, I would stop this kind of life.
>
> *(19-year-old woman, Zambia)*

While gender norms can push women into sexual relationships, they also locate the burden of responsibility onto women who become pregnant outside of marriage or of a stable long-term relationship (where paternal responsibility would more likely be assumed). A number of our participants had entered sexual-economic exchange after experiencing an early and unintended pregnancy and who had subsequently been rejected by their families who refused to support them and their infant and abandoned by the father of their child.

A 19-year-old Zimbabwean woman told us:

> We are providing for the children alone because their fathers led us to believe that they loved us and would never leave us. But once we got pregnant, they

> fled saying that they did not want to have children yet and still wanted to enjoy life as bachelors. This also left us stranded as we could not return home because our parents would not accept our pregnancies.

A similar narrative was shared in Madagascar, with one young woman reporting:

> At eighteen (years of age) my father kicked me out of our family home because he said I had dishonoured our family by becoming pregnant. So then I went to live with my aunt, but she needed me to bring money and I had no other way to support myself.
>
> *(20-year-old woman, Madagascar)*

And again in Mozambique:

> When I got involved with a boy, I got pregnant. My parents, they didn't like it. They kicked me out of the house, and I stayed with him. We had the first child, then the second, then he had an accident, he lost his life. It was when I started this life, I couldn't support the children. I noticed that my mother didn't work, my father is also disabled. I came here to Nampula to make this life.
>
> *(23-year-old woman, Mozambique)*

A number of women in Zimbabwe told us they had entered marriages at an early age which had since dissolved. The financial burden of caring for children born from these marriages was the primary responsibility of the young women with little, if any, financial support from the fathers of the children. As one 18-year-old woman explained: 'My first (child) was during my marriage and the second one, his father left me when I was pregnant. After I gave birth a friend of mine invited me to start selling sex and that is when I started until now, both my parents are deceased and this is my means of survival'.

The economy of sexual exchange is also strongly linked to family networks and lack thereof. Family networks can be seen as a modern iteration of more traditional sociocultural practices whereby families choose partners for their daughters and encourage them to start engaging in sexual relationships from an early age (Binet & Gastineau, 2008), often in return for money or cattle from the husband or partner (Mutti, 2014). The widespread social acceptance of this type of practice was reflected by comments from our participants in Madagascar, who saw it as part of "normal" life. Family involvement stems from what seems to be a widely accepted perception that parents cannot be expected to materially support their daughters above the age of 14 or 15, and these girls should then earn their own upkeep and frequently also contribute to the subsistence of the rest of the household. In some cases, we were told that families are directly responsible for finding and arranging sexual partners for their daughters in return for payment of some kind. The Madagascar case echoes our research in Zambia, which found complex interactions between the specific contexts of Zambian communities, sexual-economic exchanges, and unintended pregnancy (Zulu et al., 2024). In particular, the role of parents in enabling these relationships emerged strongly in the data. Other research in Zambia has also highlighted the economic dimension of early childbearing, which included parents encouraging their girl children to enter sexual relationships with boyfriends "to get something to eat" (Blystad et al., 2020, p. 9) and also parents arranging early marriages for their daughters in order to receive bridewealth or dowry.

In Madagascar, participants in all focus group discussions talked about examples when an older man would offer to build a house or pay a monthly fee to a family in exchange for sexual relations with their daughter, and several explicitly talked about the fact that parents would "sell" their daughters. These practices are understood as modern transformations of older traditions of arranged marriages and parents' involvement in their daughters' sexual lives, under pressure of modern economic conditions and needs of the families. In one focus group discussion, it was suggested that from the time a daughter was born, the family would be making plans for how best to economically benefit from her sexual partnerships or marriage when she was older. One respondent even evoked the fact that when a girl is born, people say of the parents that "they've had a prostitute (*prostituée*)", referring to the fact that the girl's sexuality will be a source of income for the parents when she gets older (21-year-old woman, Madagascar).

In terms of the agency of the young women involved, whilst it might be imagined that they might gain some power and independence through these sexual-economic exchanges, it was largely felt by our participants that parents were in power and controlled both their daughters' relationships and the money that they earned, thus limiting any form of emancipation or agency that might exist through these practices.

On the other hand, where households have been fractured by economic migration and/or high AIDS-related deaths, young girls are left to economically fend for themselves and often their younger siblings and/or elderly grandmothers.

> I started sex work because I am a double orphan, I don't have parents. You know how it is when you don't have parents, things are usually hard. Also there is no one to help and I had met some friends of mine who were doing the similar work, they told me about it and that's was how I joined them.
>
> *(20-year-old woman, Zambia)*

I lost my family early, and my friend started bringing me here in the city. She said: "I know a place where you can earn money. If you want to go there, we can go". People would come to talk to me, I was afraid, because I didn't know anything, it was my first day, I was afraid, I got scared, I went back home and stayed there for a week. She (the friend) always came to my house to show me money that she had earned and it gave me pain because I needed money to do many things. For example, at that moment I still went to school, yes, sometimes I didn't have money to pay tuition fees.

*(22-year-old woman, Mozambique)*

Peer networks also play an important role in introducing young women into sexual-economic exchanges and facilitating them to meet men. Peers are often instrumental in encouraging young people to have their first sexual relationship in a context where gender norms push strongly for young women and men to be in relationships from a young age and those who are not in such relationships may be stigmatised. As one young woman in Madagascar explained:

Sometimes my friends wouldn't wait for me at lunchtime, and they avoided me when we had to do group work at school because I was the only one of my group who was still a virgin.

*(16-year-old woman, Madagascar)*

Previous studies have noted the role of peer pressure and peer networks in pushing young women into relationships with "sugar daddies" (Van der Heijden and Swartz, 2014), but our findings show an even wider involvement of peers, who may encourage young women to start sexual relationships and facilitate meetings and negotiating of payment or recompense for these relationships. As one 20-year-old Zimbabwean woman explained, it was through friends that she was introduced to sexual-economic exchange:

Word of mouth through the friends I hang out with. They said that you cannot just sit around. There are many things that you can do to get money; that's how I started.

A young Madagascan woman recounted her first sexual relationship:

For my first boyfriend, it was my friends who encouraged me to have sex with him. They told me to have sex with him because he had money. My friends were doing the same thing. They were having sex with boys to get money.

The fact that their friends are involved in the same kind of sexual-economic exchange seems to act as a support mechanism for these girls and women, who find that peers are a source of information and help in managing their relationships. Again, the fact that peers are often instrumental in organising and facilitating these relationships and talk about them openly negates the argument that has been made by some that social stigma from peers is a barrier to young women accessing support or services when they are engaged in sexual-economic exchange.

An intersectional approach also helps to understand the situations of vulnerability that women find themselves in after they have become involved in sexual-economic exchange. In particular, vulnerabilities to various forms of SGBV were present for all of these young women. Often, younger age and subordinate social status were important determinants of this vulnerability to SGBV (Crankshaw et al., 2021; Freedman et al., 2021), as was a lack of legal citizenship status (as will be discussed further in the chapter) (Freedman et al., 2020b). We return to the issue of SGBV in more detail in Chapter 5.

### Identification and Structuring of Sex Work Programmes

Whilst being identified as sex workers might increase the risk of legal repercussions for women, including arrest and possible detention in countries where sex work is criminalised, we also found that being identified as a sex worker and incorporated into one of the sex work organisations which were targeted for donor funding may have advantages for some of these women but not others who may equally, if not in more vulnerable positions. In one of our study countries, for example, there is a national programme which provides much-needed clinical, mental health, and educational support services for sex workers, as well as addresses issues related to SGBV. These services are only available to self-identified sex workers. Not identifying as selling sex (even if engaged in sexual-economic exchange) precludes participation in these kinds of programmes, as they are key populations and predominantly HIV-focused and funded. And even if women self-identify as selling sex, age differentials and sex work hierarchies may deter younger women from accessing the care. Evidence in the Zimbabwean setting, for example, suggests that young women who sell sex under the age of 25, as well as those who have only recently started selling sex, may not identify as sex workers (Hensen, 2019) and are less likely to access sex work-specific services (Napierala et al., 2018).

For those women categorised as sex workers, we have noted in our research that the key population/group vulnerability approach has often led to the creation of "gatekeepers", mainly older women sex workers or previous sex workers, who have founded associations which receive funding support from different (mainly international) sources via programmes focused on identified "sex workers" and who may attempt to limit access to the group so that they can keep control of these resources, and the other advantages gained from belonging to the group. In another study country, for example, we were reprimanded by the president of a key sex worker organisation in the country for including in our interview sample young women engaged in sexual-economic exchange but who were not identified as sex workers or recognised as part of this group. She argued that her organisation was the only authorised one representing sex workers and that all research and programmes on any kind of sexual-economic exchange should pass through this organisation. We argue that this type of gatekeeping is a direct effect of the ways in which international and regional programmes on HIV have constituted "sex workers" as a key population and have defined them in a restrictive way (as discussed above). This reinforces the exclusion of women engaging in sexual-economic exchange but who are not identified as "sex workers". In poor countries, the competition for resources from this type of programme is fierce, and so there is a real interest for local organisations to maintain the strict categorisations in order to attract funding through their own networks and members. This type of gatekeeping by "established" sex workers can result in a lack of attention to power disparities between, for example, older and younger sex workers, or those from different social classes. Issues of seniority and age-related factors within sex worker hierarchies and how this impacts cohesion within the group and concomitant access to care are frequently overlooked in the literature but are highly visible on the ground. In a context of scarce resources and many young women selling sex, competition among younger and older women who sell sex is high. Our Zimbabwean research highlighted how older sex workers (>20/21 years) refused to share information about abusive clients (in order to avoid them) with younger peers, and younger women (<18/19 years) were generally distrustful of adult and older peer educators, who were also sex workers themselves (Crankshaw et al., 2021). Further, we found that very young women who self-identify as selling sex do not often access sex worker-tailored services due to age differentials and sex worker hierarchies (Crankshaw et al., 2021). Power disparities became even more visible during the global COVID-19 pandemic. In our research in Mozambique, for example, we observed how a decline in the number of clients led to the initiation of a rotational scheme in one of Maputo's main hotspots,[4] grouping sex workers according to age and alternating their days of work. Appointed "chief" sex workers, who were all older sex workers and in charge of checking scheme compliance, were found to use their position to discipline the young sex workers and turn a blind eye to their peers when working on non-allocated days (Aantjes et al., 2022b).

The notion of "intentionality" or "instrumentality" of sexual-economic exchange has been used in some research to help establish and reinforce the distinction between different categories of sex work/transactional sex. But in our research, we found that this "intentionality" was also fluid and dynamic, with women occupying a multiplicity of positions with relation to their intention to participate in and their understandings of sexual-economic exchange, which were not characterised by a clear or measurable division between "sex workers" and those involved in "transactional sex". This was also true of the degree of emotional intimacy involved in sexual relationships. Many young women who did not self-identify as sex workers stated that their primary reasons for being involved in a sexual relationship were to gain money, either for themselves or their families (Freedman et al., 2021). Others who did self-identify as sex workers had long-term affective and emotional relationships, including with men who might be described as their "clients" (Crankshaw et al., 2021). In Madagascar, for example, when we asked young women involved in sexual-economic exchange but not identifying as "sex workers" what they perceived the difference to be, they often had no answers or came up with explanations such as the fact that sex workers approached men in bars, whilst they just sat in the bars and waited for men to approach them. Such minor differences used to try and justify this differentiation seem to support the conclusion that this distinction is very blurred and not founded in real differences in women's lives and SRH outcomes but has impacts in terms of the services and support that they can access.

One of the legacies underlying this debate between the conceptual binaries of informal, relationship-based "transactional sex" versus formal or commercialised "sex work" is that of competing visions of agency and constraint for women engaging in various forms of sexual-economic exchange. In earlier literature, by presenting young women involved in "transactional sex" as exercising agency in meeting their economic and/or consumerist needs through informal sexual exchanges within relationships (Groes-Green, 2013; Masvawure, 2010; Zembe et al., 2013), there may be an implicit assumption that sex workers are, on the contrary, marginalised and victimised with little or no agency or choice. Again, we can understand these representations in colonial and gendered terms stemming from an "artificial divide" (Kapur, 2001, p. 868) between the (emancipated) sex workers in the Global North versus those in the Global South, who are consistently represented as the "disempowered victim" (Kapur, 2001, p. 857). Further, the concerns around agency in conceptualisations of transactional sex evoke the long-standing feminist debates between the abolitionist approach to sex work, which views sex work as an exploitative practice rooted within structures of patriarchy, and the pro-sex worker feminist tradition, where selling sex is argued to be a legitimate form of work and should either be legalised or decriminalised. Importantly, for the purpose of our analysis, these debates revolve around the dichotomies of victimhood and deterministic structures versus agency and self-determination, although sometimes at the expense of acknowledging the influence of context (Smith, 2011). It is plausible that faced with a population of young women involved in sexual exchanges who didn't fit post-colonial abolitionist conceptions of the stigmatised, disenfranchised "sex worker" of the Global North, the research seeking to understand the determinants of HIV in sub-Saharan Africa sought to counter the narrative of stigmatisation and victimhood and, in doing so, contributed towards the creation of a category of sexual exchange that focused explicitly on agency (and some form of emotional attachment) and therefore distanced sexual exchange practices from the traditional "sex work" paradigms. But in doing so, this research also risks reifying the idea of agency and ignoring the structural economic inequalities and violence within which sexual exchange takes place. Our research pointed to the unnecessary opposition between agency and constraint, reflecting a diversity of overlapping motives and determinants within sexual-economic exchanges that should not be considered mutually exclusive. Economic necessity strongly underpinned sexual exchanges in all of our research settings, but there also existed an element of consumerist-driven motivations or aspirations for social mobility. And while young women – whether they identify as selling sex or not – exercise varying degrees of agency, this agency is constrained by an overarching structural context where the dynamics of unequal gender, age, and economic power relations play out in ways that create particular vulnerability for poor SRH outcomes. Rather than agency being placed at odds with structures of vulnerability, we argue for an approach where 'structure is treated as mutually constitutive of agency' (Smith, 2011, p. 539).

Rather than continue to engage in polarising debates over conceptual differences between commercial sex work and transactional sex and to oppose essentialised and monolithic views of agency versus victimhood, we argue for an approach which recognises the situated intersectionalities leading to various vulnerabilities which need to be addressed. Following feminist theorists such as Fineman (2017), we argue for the use of vulnerability understood not as linked with categories or group identities but as fluid and as determined by an individual's position within different social structures. This implies responsibilities on the part of the state to address these structural inequalities to increase resilience, understood as an individual's capacity to take advantage of opportunities and cope with adversity (Fineman, 2017). If unequal access to societal structures or unequal allocations of privilege and power within social structures diminish resilience (Fineman, 2017), then we can argue that we need to address these unequal allocations to ensure rights and justice for all. This approach would allow us to better understand the reasons for young women's engagement in these exchanges, the meanings that they and their families and peers give to them, and the resulting conditions of vulnerability or violence which emerge from them.

## Sexual-Economic Exchange in the Context of Forced Displacement

In our research in Madagascar, Mozambique, Zambia, and Zimbabwe discussed above, we found that there were various intersecting inequalities which led to women's involvement in sexual-economic exchange and which reinforced their situations of vulnerability within these exchanges. An additional axis of inequality which has a huge impact on women's situation is that of their legal residence or citizenship status. This was shown clearly in our research amongst young refugee women living in South Africa, where they described a variety of sexual-economic relationships underpinned by legal and economic insecurity.

For these young women, engagement in sexual-economic exchange had often begun on their journey to escape their countries of origin and flee to South Africa. Frequently, they told us they did not have money for transport and were thus forced to bargain with truck drivers to give them a ride to their destination. Gendered expectations around (men's) assistance repaid in the form of (women's) sexual exchange were the norm for drivers or smugglers helping women reach South Africa. However, there also existed a coercive element where women had to comply or risk being left stranded in highly insecure conflict or unknown contexts, as the following woman refugee recounted:

> Like the journey most of the women that we were with……you know, because there was someone who was conducting us to come here. There was like a leader who was leading us to come to South Africa because for us we didn't know the way. So that man used to like take women to sleep with them to help them with food or just to help them to take them to their journey. Some of them were not accepting, but I know that for those ones that would refuse, he left them there. Like some were left by the border in Zimbabwe, Zambia, and some they got arrested.
>
> *(24-year-old Congolese woman, South Africa)*

These women were afforded no safe refuge upon arriving in South Africa, finding themselves in extremely vulnerable situations with no legal papers, little money, and usually not speaking a local language. A 24-year-old woman, born to a Zambian mother and Congolese father, explained that when she arrived in South Africa, the truck drivers who had brought her dropped her in Johannesburg (an inland city in South Africa) rather than Durban (approximately 570 km away from Johannesburg), as they had promised. She found herself stranded at the bus station in Johannesburg, with no money and unable to understand how she could travel onwards:

> That's when I was stranded. I reached the bus station. I didn't have any money and my phone was off (battery was flat). I stayed there and then

> another guy who was waiting there, he was like 'You've stayed here for a long time. Why? What are you waiting for?'. It was even getting dark. And I said, I don't have anywhere to go, or anyone to help me to reach where I'm going. And so that guy told me 'No, let's go to my house. You can charge your phone, then call your people to send your money'. So that's when I followed that guy to his place. Then he told me to sit down. He gave me juice. Then I took the juice and he was like, 'How old are you?' Then I told him that I was 20 years old. 'So do you have a boyfriend?' and I said no I don't have a boyfriend. And he said 'I'm interested in you'. I said 'No, no I'm not interested. I didn't come for those things'. Then he told me: 'How are you going to get help if you don't want this thing?' And I was just confused. Then he told me that it was getting dark and he said: 'Are you going to sleep here or what? Or you are going now? Should I open the door for you?' And I was like, No, I don't have anywhere to go. And people have told me it's dangerous around here. So that's when he told me. 'That's okay. If you want me to help you, then sleep with me, I'll give you the money for the transport to go wherever you want to go'.

The man kept sending messages to this young woman once she had reached Durban and asked her to come back to see him again in Johannesburg. But when she did go back, she found he was in a relationship with another woman, and as she says found herself "stranded" again, and had to accept sex with a truck driver to get back to Durban.

Refugee women seeking refugee protection find it difficult to obtain legal status due to barriers within the asylum system (Crankshaw et al., 2023; Mutambara et al., 2023). This leaves them in vulnerable situations, where they also find it difficult to obtain work, as one 25-year-old Congolese woman recounts:

> And after that I started to look for a job. I did an interview and then they checked my (asylum) paper. It was almost expired, only a few days were left. They said, I could go back to Home Affairs and renew. And then come back and they'd give me the job. I went to renew. I was even praying. I first say, God, I need this job. Then I came back to the office. I found the manager. I told her I'd already done the interview. And they said I already got the job. But what was needed is just to renew my papers. So I showed her my new papers. And then she said, No, we don't take people that have that type of paper, because my paper was for six months, I had to renew it every six months. So I was feeling very, very, very disappointed.

This young woman then entered into a sexual relationship with a foreigner living nearby. As she explains:

> He's a white guy. He's very old, 64 years old. He told me that he's married but he needs someone for "intimacy" things. Because him and his wife have a problem on that side. And so for me, because I need this money to survive and feed my child, I said, okay, no problem.

Barriers to gaining employment mean that women have to rely on the informal sector, where they are subject to exploitation. Many women spoke about the fact that even when they did find some kind of work, it was insufficient to meet their needs and those of their families. This echoes the findings from other countries (see above), where women recounted engaging in sexual-economic exchanges in addition to other forms of employment.

This lack of employment contributes to situations of economic insecurity where women have little choice other than to engage in sexual relationships to provide for themselves and their children:

> Yeah, yeah, I have been in so many relationships like that because I just need money for my kids, like maybe sometimes if the baby – there is no milk, there is no food – starts crying. There's nothing in the house. Maybe you think of a guy that was disturbing you and you just call him and yeah.
>
> *(24-year-old Congolese woman, South Africa)*

> Because you find yourself without any support, but there's a guy there outside who says now I'm ready to help you. So what you're gonna do? Like, as we don't have money to pay rent, you need money to pay the rent, and then you find out there is a guy outside, they're going to help you to pay those things. You can't say no, because you need it.
>
> *(23-year-old Congolese woman, South Africa)*

Lack of housing also placed women in situations of vulnerability (refugees receive no state aid or help in finding housing in South Africa). Women told us that they had entered into sexual relationships, either short or long term, in order to find somewhere to sleep off the streets.

> For myself, I don't know, because, you know, here there's no family. The things that send us to do such things (engage in sexual-economic exchanges)

> is because today we don't have money to pay rent. We stay on the street. So that's why maybe for me, myself doing this, because I know I have to pay the rent because (the landlord) chased me for the first time. They chased me because I didn't have a job or money to pay rent, so they put me outside. I was outside. So I just scored a big guy. So which means if that guy didn't have a place (to live), maybe I could be on the street, right?
>
> *(25-year-old Congolese woman, South Africa)*

The extreme vulnerability of these young women meant that they had little or no power within sexual relationships and were unable to negotiate condom use. A number of women recounted that they had subsequently discovered they had acquired HIV.

> Some of them do use protection, and some of them do not want to use it, but you know that we need the money. So even if they say they don't want (to use a condom), at the end of the day, they don't want it, But if you tell them that you don't want it and you need to pay (expenses), if they say yes, yes. If they say no, then no.
>
> *(22-year-old Congolese woman, South Africa)*

Dependency also leads to women remaining in relationships where they experience violence. Several of the women recounted that their partners would come home drunk and then beat them, but they could not leave because they had nowhere else to go. This links to our discussions of the vulnerabilities of refugee women to SGBV in Chapter 5 of this book. The relationships were not viewed merely as "transactional", however, emphasising the continuum between different forms of sexual exchanges, which can involve affection and emotion, and looking for someone to "take care" of them. One young woman explained:

> A lot of foreigners (refugees), they do these things because they will be struggling with kids, and they usually do not have any support from their baby daddies. So, you end up selling yourself just for money. Not like that thing of standing on the side of the road waiting for someone to come and pick you up for sex, but more like entering a relationship for money, wanting the person to take care of you.
>
> *(23-year-old Congolese woman, South Africa)*

This feeling of needing to be "taken care of" was reinforced by the fact that being a refugee in South Africa meant that these women often felt very isolated and far away from any friends or family who could support them. This meant that they looked for love and support in these sexual-economic exchanges. This isolation also reinforced their dependency once in a relationship. One woman who had been homeless and had entered into a sexual relationship with a man to get off the streets, told us that she now felt trapped:

> I thought that when I met up with this man, things will be kind of easier for me. But now things are getting worse for me. Like now I have two kids and when I think about leaving, or going to another country, how am I even going to go because I came to South Africa when I was really small. I do not know who's in Congo. I don't even talk with any of my family members.
>
> *(22-year-old Congolese woman, South Africa)*

Marriage was often viewed as a way to provide economic security in all our research contexts, including amongst young women who self-identified as selling sex and also in a context where refugees have very limited legal rights and economic opportunities, with parents (should they be present) playing a strong role in arranging these unions. This draws parallels with what we found in our research in Madagascar and Zambia concerning the role of parents in arranging sexual partnerships for their daughters.

> It's not like you want to. And, you know, sometimes your parents put pressure on you, if you are the type that says I should obey my parent … You just find out like when you are married, you are not actually happy because it's not that you wanted to. This is just something that you do for the sake of getting out of the lifestyle and the situation that you've been through.
>
> *(19-year-old Congolese woman, South Africa)*

> They are using marriage as a way or method of getting money back in the family. The biggest challenge we have is forced marriages.
>
> *(18-year-old Congolese woman, South Africa)*

## Conclusions

In her analysis of the commodification of sex in SSA, Ampofo notes that 'the social organisation (sic) of sexual exchange takes a variety of forms in different historical and cultural contexts and political economies so that we cannot speak of any universal form' (Ampofo, 2001, p. 27). In this chapter, we have sought to make a case to move away from categorical labels and dichotomies between "sex work" and "transactional sex" and to move towards an approach which understands situated vulnerabilities for young women based on their positioning within varied axes of structural inequalities. Whether defined as sex workers or not, these young women face situations of insecurity, vulnerability to violence, and poor SRHR. We argue that moving from a public health approach centred on

HIV risk and a perceived need to measure different forms of sexual-economic exchange in order to quantify this risk and towards an approach which emphasises instead a holistic concern for women's sexual and reproductive health would be a step forward in strengthening their rights. Current programmes or policies which target either "sex workers" or women involved in "transactional sex" may lead to fragmentation and an overlooking of the situations and determinants of vulnerability which are common to all, particularly so for younger women. Rather, we argue for policies and programmes which take into account the various structural and proximate factors which constrain young women's sexual choices and which expose them to various situations of vulnerability as a result. Considering the broader context of structures of poverty, gender inequality, and inequalities based on age, ethnicity, citizenship, and legal status, among others, with the goal of improving young women's sexual and reproductive health and rights more generally, this could be a step in the direction of realising those rights.

## Notes

1 We use the term continuum in the same sense here as that used to describe a "continuum of violence" (Kelly, 198: p.76), and that we will discuss more fully in Chapter 5. In other words, various forms of sexual-economic exchange can all be linked to their foundation in underlying structural inequalities and seen as 'a continuous series of elements or events that pass into one another and cannot be readily distinguished'.

2 Interestingly, despite providing this operational definition, the same UNAIDS document underscores the need to 'develop accurate definitions of the wide range of transactional sex behaviors involved' and in their subsequent Technical Update on Sex Work and HIV AIDS (2002) define sex workers as 'female, male and transgender adults and young people who receive money or goods in exchange for sexual services, either regularly or occasionally, and who may or may not consciously define those activities as income-generating' (UNAIDS, 2002, p. 3).

3 Section 61 of the Criminal Code defines a "prostitute" to mean 'a male or female person who for money or reward: (a) allows other persons to have anal or extra-marital sexual intercourse or engage in other sexual conduct with him or her; or (b) solicits other persons to have anal or extra-marital sexual intercourse or engage in other sexual conduct with him or her'.

4 The term hotspot refers to areas within downtown cities, around ports, along main truck routes and border posts where sex workers solicit clients on the street or in bars.

## References

Aantjes, C., Crankshaw, T. L., & Freedman, J. (2022a). Impacts of colonial legacies on the rights and security of sex workers in Southern Africa. *International Journal of Gender, Sexuality and Law*, *2*(1), 273–297.

Aantjes, C., Muchanga, V., & Munguambe, K. (2022b). Exposed and unprotected: Sex workers vulnerabilities during the COVID-19 health emergency in Mozambique. *Global Public Health*, *17*, 3568–3582.

Akin-Aina, S. (2011). Beyond an epistemology of bread, butter, culture and power: Mapping the African feminist movement. *Nokoko*, *2*, 65–89.

Ampofo, A. A. (2001). The sex trade, globalisation and issues of survival in sub-Saharan Africa. *Institute of African Studies Research Review*, *17*(2), 27–43.

Anderson, E. L. (2015). *Gender, HIV and risk: Navigating structural violence*. Palgrave Macmillan.

Ankomah, A. (1999). Sex, love, money and AIDS: The dynamics of premarital sexual relationships in Ghana. *Sexualities*, *2*(3), 291–308.

Binet, C., & Gastineau, B. (2008). Marriage, fecundity, and conjugal autonomy in Madagascar. *Autrepart*, *47*(3), 43–56.

Blystad, A., Moland, K. M., Munsaka, E., Sandøy, I., & Zulu, J. (2020). Vanilla bisquits and lobola bridewealth: Parallel discourses on early pregnancy and schooling in rural Zambia. *BMC Public Health*, *20*, 1–11.

Cole, J. (2004). Fresh contact in Tamatave, Madagascar: Sex, money, and intergenerational transformation. *American Ethnologist*, *31*(4), 573–588.

Cole, J. (2009). Love, money, and economies of intimacy in Tamatave, Madagascar. In J. Cole, & L. M. Thomas (Eds.), *Love in Africa* (pp. 109–134, 2009. Chicago Scholarship Online, pages). University of Chicago Press.

Crankshaw, T. L., Chareka, S., Zambezi, P., & Poku, N. K. (2021). Age matters: Determinants of sexual and reproductive health vulnerabilities amongst young women who sell sex (16–24 years) in Zimbabwe. *Social Science and Medicine*, *270*, 113597.

Crankshaw, T. L., & Freedman, J. (2023). Sex work or transactional sex? Shifting the dialogue from risk to rights. *Sexual and Reproductive Health Matters*, *31*(1), 1–9.

Crankshaw, T. L., Freedman, J., & Mutambara, V. M. (2023). Intergenerational trajectories of inherited vulnerabilities amongst young women refugees in South Africa. *Comparative Migration Studies*, *11*(1), 1–18.

Dellar, R. C., Dlamini, S., & Karim, Q. A. (2015). Adolescent girls and young women: Key populations for HIV epidemic control. *Journal of the International AIDS Society*, *18*, 19408.

Ditmore, M. H., & Allman, D. (2013). An analysis of the implementation of PEPFAR's anti-prostitution pledge and its implications for successful HIV prevention among organisations working with sex Workers. *Journal of the International AIDS Society*, *16*(1), 17354.

Fineman, M. (2017). Vulnerability and inevitable inequality. *Oslo Law Review*, *4*(3), 133–149.

Flint, V., & Hewitt, V. (2015). Colonial tropes and HIV/AIDS in Africa: Sex, disease and race. *Commonwealth & Comparative Politics*, *53*(3), 294–314.

Formson, C., & Hilhorst, D. (2016). *The many faces of transactional sex: Women's agency, livelihoods and risk factors in humanitarian contexts*. Wageningen University.

Freedman, J., Crankshaw, T. L., & Mutambara, V. M. (2020b). Sexual and reproductive health of asylum seeking and refugee women in South Africa: Understanding the determinants of vulnerability. *Sexual and Reproductive Health Matters*, *28*(1), 1758440.

Freedman, J., Rakotoarindrasata, M., & de Dieu Randrianasolorivo, J. (2021). Analysing the economies of transactional sex amongst young people: Case study of Madagascar. *World Development*, *138*, 105289.

Freedman, J., Rakotoarindrasata, M., & de Dieu Randrianasolorivo, J. (2020a). *Remise en cause des frontières supposées entre travail du sexe et sexe transactionnel à Madagascar-le cas de Nosy-be. Institut du Genre en Géopolitique*.

Groes-Green, C. (2013). "To put men in a bottle": Eroticism, kinship, female power, and transactional sex in Maputo, Mozambique. *American Ethnologist*, *40*(1), 102–117.

Hensen, B., Chabata, S. T., Floyd, S., Chiyaka, T., Mushati, P., Busza, J., Birdthistle, I., Hargreaves, J. R., & Cowan, F. M. (2019). HIV risk among young women who sell sex by whether they identify as sex workers: Analysis of respondent-driven sampling surveys, Zimbabwe, 2017. *Journal of International AIDS Society*, *22*(12), e25410.

Hill, D. (2020). *'Damage and Womanhood in the Lives of Female Prostitutes in Zambia'*. Unpublished doctoral thesis, University of Sussex.

Hunter, M. (2002). The materiality of everyday sex: Thinking beyond prostitution. *Journal of Africa Studies*, *61*(1), 99–120.

Kapur, R. (2001). Post-colonial economies of desire: Legal representations of the Sexual Subaltern. *Denver University Law Review*, *78*, 855.

Maganja, R. K., Maman, S., Groves, A., & Mbwambo, J. K. (2007). Skinning the goat and pulling the load: Transactional sex among youth in Dar es Salaam, Tanzania. *AIDS Care*, *19*(8), 974–981.

Masvawure, T. (2010). 'I just need to be flashy on campus': Female students and transactional sex at a university in Zimbabwe. *Culture, Health & Sexuality*, *12*(8), 857–870.

McMillan, K., Worth, H., & Rawstorne, P. (2018). Usage of the terms prostitution, sex work, transactional sex, and survival sex: Their utility in HIV prevention research. *Archives of Sexual Behavior*, *47*(5), 1517–1527.

Merten, S., & Haller, T. (2007). Culture, changing livelihoods, and HIV/AIDS discourse: Reframing the institutionalization of fish-for-sex exchange in the Zambian Kafue Flats. *Culture, Health & Sexuality*, *9*(1), 69–83.

Mgbako, C. A. (2016). *To live freely in this world: Sex worker activism in Africa*. NYU Press.

Mgbako, C., & Smith, L. A. (2009). Sex work and human rights in Africa. *Fordham International Law Journal*, *33*(4), 1178–1220.

Mutambara, V. M., Crankshaw, T. L., & Freedman, J. (2022). Assessing the impacts of COVID-19 on women refugees in South Africa. *Journal of Refugee Studies*, *35*(1), 704–721.

Mutambara, V. M., Freedman, J., Crankshaw, T. L., & Rajah, Y. (2023). Gendered insecurities: Exploring the continuum of sexual and gender-based violence experiences of refugee women in South Africa. In *The Gender of Borders* (pp. 103–118). Routledge.

Mutti, V. A. (2014). Et les garçons? reflections on Unicef Program for girls post primary education in Madagascar. In African Dynamics in a Multipolar World: 5th European Conference on African Studies—Conference Proceedings (pp. 1484–1499). Centro de Estudos Internacionais do Instituto Universitário de Lisboa (ISCTE-IUL).

Napierala, S., Chabata, S. T., Fearon, E., Davey, C., Hargreaves, J., Busza, J., Mushati, P., Mtetwa, S., Chiyaka, T., Mugurungi, O., Hanisch, D., Hatzold, K., Phillips, A., Cowan, F. M. (2018). Engagement in HIV care among young female sex workers in Zimbabwe. *JAIDS Journal of Acquired Immune Deficiency Syndromes*, *79*(3), 358–366.

Ndlovu-Gatsheni, S. J. (2013). *Coloniality of power in postcolonial Africa*. African Books Collective.

Richter, M. (2012). Sex work as a test case for African feminism. *A Journal on African Women's Experiences*, *2*(1), 62–69.

Schoepf, B. G. (1988). Women, AIDS, and economic crisis in Central Africa. *Canadian Journal of African Studies/La Revue canadienne des études africaines*, *22*(3), 625–644.

Smith, N. J. (2011). The international political economy of commercial sex. *Review of International Political Economy*, *18*(4), 530–549.

Stoebenau, K., Heise, L., Wamoyi, J., & Bobrova, N. (2016). Revisiting the understanding of "transactional sex" in sub-Saharan Africa: A review and synthesis of the literature. *Social Science & Medicine*, *168*, 186–197.

Tabet, P. (2005). La grande arnaque: sexualité des femmes et échange économico-sexuel. *La grande arnaque*, 1–211.

Tabet, P. (2012). Through the looking-glass: sexual-economic exchange. *Chic, Cheque, Choc. Transactions autor des corps et stratégies amoureuses*, 39–51.
The Lancet. (2022). PEPFAR looks to the future. *The lancet. HIV*, *9*(6), e367.
UNAIDS. (2000). *Regional Workshop on Situation Analysis of Sex Work in West and Central Africa* Abidjan, 21–24 March 2000, Cote d'Ivoire.
UNAIDS. (2002). *Technical update sex work and HIV/AIDS*. UNAIDS.
UNAIDS. (2018). *Transactional sex and HIV risk: From analysis to action*. Joint United Nations Programme on HIV/AIDS and STRIVE.
UNAIDS. (2022). *UNAIDS global AIDS update 2022*. UNAIDS.
van der Heijden, I., & Swartz, S. (2014). 'Something for something': The importance of talking about transactional sex with youth in South Africa using a resilience-based approach. *African Journal of Agricultural Research, 13*(1), 53–63.
Wamoyi, J., Ranganathan, M., Kyegombe, N., & Stoebenau, K. (2019). Improving the measurement of transactional sex in Sub-Saharan Africa: A critical review. *JAIDS Journal of Acquired Immune Deficiency Syndromes*, *80*(4), 367–374.
White, S. K., & Kamya, H. A. (2022). Transactional sex, consumer society, and neoliberalism in Uganda: A political economic analysis of drivers and models of response. *Global Public Health*, *17*(7), 1343–1357.
World Health Organisation. (2015). *Technical brief: HIV and young people who sell sex*. WHO.
Yuval-Davis, N. (2015). Situated intersectionality and social inequality. *Raisons Politiques*, 58, 91–100.
Zembe, Y. Z., Townsend, L., Thorson, A., & Ekström, A. M. (2013). "Money talks, bullshit walks" interrogating notions of consumption and survival sex among young women engaging in transactional sex in post-apartheid South Africa: A qualitative enquiry. *Globalization and Health*, *9*, 1–16.
Zulu, J. Crankshaw, T.L, Ouedraogo, R., Juma, K., Aantjes, C.J. (2024). The ones at the bottom of the food chain: Structural drivers of unintended pregnancy and unsafe abortion amongst adolescent girls in Zambia., *Archives of Public Health, 82*, 1–13.

# 4

# GOING BEYOND HIV

## Shifting the Dialogue from Risk to Rights

### Introduction

The global response to the HIV and AIDS pandemic has been unprecedented in terms of the sheer amount of funding and life-saving medications being directed to the country's worst affected, but with limited means to address the scale of the challenges. Enormous progress has been made in tackling the pandemic, most notably towards the elimination of mother-to-child HIV transmission, increases in the numbers of people living with HIV initiated on treatment, and fewer deaths from AIDS-related illness. A closer analysis, however, reveals that much of the headway has been made in the *treatment* of AIDS rather than preventing HIV infection from occurring in the first place. The reality is that HIV prevention is lagging woefully behind, and this is evident in the ongoing high rates of new HIV infections. The period between 2020 and 2021 saw the smallest annual decline in new HIV infections globally since 2016, and there is indication that new infections are rising rapidly. Young women continue to bear the burden of new HIV infections. Sixty-three percent of all new HIV infections in 2021 were amongst women and girls (UNAIDS, 2022), and girls account for six in seven new HIV infections among adolescents aged 15–19 years. Eastern and Southern Africa (ESA) is a region that is disproportionately burdened by HIV. In 2019, 43% of new worldwide infections occurred in the region, which is home to an estimated 54% of all people living with HIV worldwide (Risher et al., 2021). The need to channel international funding and to move rapidly in the early days of the HIV response in countries with high HIV burdens and weak health systems has resulted in the establishment of vertical HIV programmes. And while there has long been a

DOI: 10.4324/9781003414698-4

call for the integration of HIV and other aspects of SRH, the HIV community remains mostly siloed from the SRHR community, and this is often driven by funder priorities. In this chapter, we will first trace a brief history of the HIV and AIDS response, pointing to the emergence of the "key population" approach and the way in which the use of the concept of vulnerability has been used within this approach. We will then go on to analyse the ways in which a focus on HIV and AIDS might have led to the detachment of other key SRHR issues for young women, such as access to contraception or safe abortion care. We will draw on our primary research to contextualise and reposition HIV as one of a number of SRH indicators and highlight other equally important aspects of poor SRH arising from particular intersections of vulnerability. In doing so, we will make a case for paying attention to the broader basket of SRHR issues – including HIV – which we will argue simultaneously serve to strengthen HIV prevention efforts and examine vulnerability rather than risk when targeting SRH interventions.

## What's in a Definition?: "Key Populations" and "Other Vulnerable Groups"

The term "key population" emerged over 20 years ago to identify populations that were considered "key" to the HIV epidemic dynamics and epidemic response in terms of being more likely to become infected with HIV. This has, in part, led to 'preoccupation with changing so-called "risky behaviours" of "high-risk" or "at-risk" groups or "key populations" because, with the constraints of insufficient resources, this is deemed "cost-effective". However, in doing so it implies that risk is something that is contained within these groups' (Anderson, 2015, p. 7). We will explore how these dynamics also played into the prioritisation of the treatment agenda over prevention further on in the chapter. The UN agencies define key populations as 'gay men and other men who have sex with men, sex workers, transgender people, people who inject drugs and prisoners and other incarcerated people as the five main key population groups that are particularly vulnerable to HIV and frequently lack adequate access to services'.[1] The Global Fund, which is the leading external funder of key population programmes, links the concept of key populations to three key health challenges – HIV, tuberculosis, and malaria – and understands key populations as those who 'experience both increased impact from one or more of the diseases [ie HIV, tuberculosis and/or malaria] and decreased access to services. Widespread stigma and discrimination, state and non-state violence and harassment, restrictive laws and policies, and criminalization of behaviors (sic) or practices put key populations at heightened risks and undermine their access to services'.[2] While this definition includes other infectious diseases, key populations are still largely defined in the context of HIV and include men who have sex with men, transgender people, but especially transgender women, sex workers, people who inject drugs, people living with HIV, and people in prison and detention.

Importantly, understandings of key populations have evolved – and been contested – over time. For example, in its 2022 Global AIDS Update report, UNAIDS presented statistics on new HIV infections amongst members of key population groups[3] *and* their sexual partners. On the other hand, the Global Fund has more recently included "key populations" in the context of malaria and includes refugees, migrants, internally displaced people, and indigenous populations in malaria-endemic areas who, the Global Fund states, are at greater risk of transmission; are likely to have decreased access to care and services; and are also often marginalised. Interestingly, the Global Fund also recognises "vulnerable populations" as 'those who have increased vulnerabilities in a particular context, but may not fit the criteria' of the other key population groups. Vulnerable populations are here defined as including adolescent girls and young women, and people with disabilities, among others. Interestingly, these broader definitions are strongly contested in some quarters, including amongst representatives of multilateral global health organisations who argue around the need to clearly differentiate between "key populations" and "vulnerable populations" on the basis that using broader terminologies results in key populations being hidden in the "rhetoric" of the general population, with the result that their particular needs do not come into proper focus. There is also the reality that large funders, in the face of declining external financial assistance, make decisions to fund countries on the basis of the highest proportion of "key populations" in a given area. The use of definitions and categorisations such as "key population" can thus be seen not only as health-related but also closely linked to political and economic decision-making and thus open to variations depending on those who have influence in funding decisions.

Whilst we might criticise the way that the concept of "key populations" is used today, particularly in the African context, and the impact that this usage has on progressing SRHR, historically, the focus on "key populations" has not been unjustified given the disproportionate burden of HIV and AIDS amongst the groups so defined. At the onset of the pandemic, HIV incidence was higher amongst men who have sex with men in the United States than amongst women (Merson et al., 2008), and when HIV was newly identified in 1981, it was believed by the Centers for Disease Control in the United States that the virus (Pneumocystis jirovecii) only occurred amongst men who have sex with men and that it was contained in the United States. It was only at the end of the same year that cases were also being reported in heterosexual injecting drug users and outside of the United States. Gay communities in the Global North were at the vanguard of the social movements driving accountability in the global AIDS response (Parker, 2011). Indeed, the effective mobilisation and activism around the AIDS response have been traced back to the struggle for gay liberation amongst predominantly white middle-class men in the 1970s in industrialised Western nations (Parker, 2011). However, even very early in the epidemic, tensions quickly emerged between the 'more well-to-do populations and communities affected by HIV and AIDS – particularly white gay men – and other, more marginalized (sic) populations' – including women and the poor (Parker, 2011, p. 25). As Watkins-Hayes (2014) argues with regard to early political mobilisation around HIV and AIDS in the United States, 'The ability to couple aggressive political mobilization (sic) with economic capital, highly resourced social networks, and the authority bestowed through racial privilege translated into focused attention on the challenges faced by (mostly) white gay middle-class men and exposed deep societal homophobia. However, their stories came overwhelmingly to represent the universal experience of HIV/AIDS (sic), marginalizing (sic) the struggles of other groups who were having different experiences by virtue of race, gender, class, and sexuality' (Watkins-Hayes, 2014, p. 450). It is important to understand this historical context since these dynamics also shaped the global narrative, with the 'more narrow focus of determined treatment activists in the global North intent on changing the system to gain access to life-saving medications [which] often came into conflict with a broader set of concerns about the structural conditions that placed more marginalized (sic) populations at increased vulnerability' (Parker, 2011, p. 26). Our research investigating the economic, social, and health impacts of COVID-19 on young people of diverse genders and sexualities who sell sex in Zimbabwe, for example, found that vulnerability was unequally distributed by geography and socio-economic position, as well as by gender, sex, and age, both within and between "key population" groups of participants (Crankshaw et al., 2023). Transgender and cisgender women faced greater sexual harassment and exploitation, and cisgender women were often living as heads of households with child dependents, which exacerbated food insecurity and influenced their ability to negotiate protected sex regardless of condom availability. Compared to many of the cisgender women participants who reported having dropped out of school, transgender and male participants were generally better educated or still studying. Most female participants relied on selling sex as their main source of income, while most male participants only engaged in sex work part-time and had other financially viable "side hustles" (Ibid.). Findings such as these strongly challenge the boundaries of the key population categorisations in the context of SRHR more holistically.

Although their scope has rapidly expanded in the era of the SDGs, a significant proportion of civil society involved in SRHR continues to be predominantly HIV-centric, with a strong continued focus on "key population" groups. We argue that the interaction of these legacies has fundamentally shaped the way that vulnerability to poor SRH (including HIV) is still understood in terms of "HIV risk" and from a predominantly male-centric perspective. As Heywood (2020) asserts, civil society has itself not fully transformed and remains a 'mirror of patriarchal society', where men predominantly lead NGOs and social movements, and that the 'outlook of male dominated leadership is reflected in both the strategies and methods of civil society' (p. 309) even though women are volunteers or form part of the organisations. Heywood writes on civil society in the South African setting, arguing that neglect of key reproductive rights issues such as contraception and abortion is a demonstration that civil society has failed to take gender equality seriously 'either as a core component of social justice or as a principle for leadership with the human rights movement' (p. 308). Given the deep experience and maturity of civil society organisations and social movements in South Africa, similar analyses need to be applied to civil society more broadly in the Southern African region. Greater engagement with continental, regional, and country-level civil society on the SRHR priorities of different populations in the roll out of people-centric, integrated SRHR care across the life-course will be important to breaking out of these silos.

Forty years later, the argument for retaining "key population" categories on the surface appears to hold strong. In 2021, key populations (which make up less than 5% of the global population) and their sexual partners accounted for 70% of HIV infections globally (UNAIDS 2022). However, this position obscures the inherent gender bias within these categorisations and fundamentally ignores contextual variations in HIV epidemic dynamics. For example, the 2023 UNAIDS Global AIDS Update identifies that women are an overlooked group *even within* the classic "key population" categories (UNAIDS, 2023). Programmes for people who use drugs, for example, have been criticised for not being responsive to the needs of women who inject drugs because globally the majority of people who inject drugs are men (Iversen et al., 2015). Moreover, there are key geopolitical differences in the burden of new HIV infections, as evident in the global trends. The character and face of the epidemic in Southern Africa is (and has always been) fundamentally different in terms of age, gender, and sexual orientation (i.e., very young women's engagement in deeply unequal heterosexual-economic exchanges) in a context of high economic inequalities and where sexual and gender-based violence is the norm. While these facts are acknowledged by those working in the HIV space, there remains an unwillingness to relinquish the idea of key population groups, defined as "key" at a global level, even in regions where these may not apply. For example, outside of sub-Saharan Africa, 94% of new HIV infections occurred amongst "key populations" and their sexual partners, with only 6% of new infections amongst the remaining population (UNAIDS 2022). However, in sub-Saharan Africa, new HIV infections were roughly balanced between "key populations" and their sexual partners (51%), and the remaining population (49%). There are also clear differences between gender and sexuality in rates of new infections between SSA and the rest of the world. Of the new infections amongst key populations in SSA, 15% were amongst sex workers and only 6% amongst gay men and other men who have sex with men. The opposite was true for the rest of the world with 41% of new infections occurring amongst gay men and other men who have sex with men, and 9% were amongst sex workers. Even though the transmission dynamics of the HIV epidemic in SSA has always differed from that of the Global North, the reality is that affected women (with limited educational and economic resources and commonly living with child dependents from a very young age) do not and have never held the same political power and influence over the global agenda in the same way as gay men from affected communities in the Global North. Instead, the situation of adolescent girls and young women can arguably be characterised by the *absence* of a social movement, as they are a diverse and widespread population largely without the economic and political power to effectively mobilise.

## The Feminisation of HIV and AIDS

We have argued about the way in which the global HIV and AIDS response was shaped by the activism and experiences of gay men in the United States. However, there has also been a push by some scholars to highlight the experiences of women in sub-Saharan Africa who have been the most affected, leading to what some researchers have called a "feminisation" of HIV and AIDS. Harman argues that in the early 2000s, with the crisis of AIDS-related deaths in sub-Saharan Africa, it became clear that women and girls were at higher risk of contracting the virus, and this led to a "feminisation" (Harman, 2011) of analyses and responses to the pandemic. In her article on this phenomenon of feminisation, Harman (2011) describes how the statistics on infection and prevalence rates, which showed that proportionally many more women than men were being infected with HIV, led governments, international organisations, NGOs, and donors to prioritise responses that focused on women and girls as a key part of the global response to the problem. Early research and analyses focused on women's biological vulnerability – the physiological differences between women's and men's bodies which make the female body more likely to be infected with HIV during heterosexual vaginal sex (Ramjee & Daniels, 2013) – ignoring the social and systemic drivers of HIV infection. We can argue that this focus on biological "causes" of greater risk of infection for women has turned attention away from wider gender inequalities – economic, political, and social – which place women in situations of vulnerability and mean that they have fewer resources to improve their resilience both to HIV and to the long-term and wider impacts of living with HIV, for example, their household as they take in and care for sick family members (Harrison et al., 2014; Hosegood et al., 2007). As Harman (2011, p. 215) asserts, 'The structural socio-economic inequalities that underpin high prevalence rates and the burden of care apportioned to women make the feminisation of HIV and AIDS more about gender and less about female biology'.

In another sense, some have described how HIV and AIDS governance also became "feminised" as international organisations and NGOs positioned women as central to the HIV and AIDS response. A focus on community-based responses to HIV and AIDS has also centralised women's role, as it is frequently women's groups within communities who have been selected as local community partners for larger national and international programmes. However, as argued above with regard to the leadership of civil society and NGOs, men generally retain the central roles and those with decision-making power, whilst 'women within the primary community continue to be pigeon-holed into positions of implementation, care and primary education, and are only able to gain leverage in decision-making by reasserting their caring function and close links with the community' (Harman, 2011, p. 221). Moreover, within international governance, individuals and organisations which prioritise a true gendered approach have tended to be sidelined (Harman, 2011). As Harman concludes, the reason that the feminisation of HIV and AIDS governance does not lead to better outcomes for women is that 'women do not necessarily make policy by virtue of their gender, and those that do recognise gender tend to be side-lined. The international organisations, states and non-governmental actors that promote inclusion as the principal mechanism of combatting the feminisation of HIV and AIDS fail to recognise this, and as such continue to perpetuate the idea that inclusion of women is enough. Thus, it is both the type of inclusion and the emphasis upon inclusion alone that makes the feminisation of HIV and AIDS particularly problematic' (Harman, 2011, p. 225).

## Colonialism and Securitisation of HIV and AIDS

As we have argued elsewhere in this book (see, for example, the discussion on sexual economic exchanges in Chapter 3), international approaches to and framings of health issues impacting Africa can be understood in the context of continuing colonialist understandings, which in turn will have an impact on how policies are designed at international, regional, and national levels. Flint and Hewitt (2015) argue that whilst HIV and AIDS were new diseases for Africa, the discourses framing them were derivative and a continuation of past colonial approaches to public health and governance on the continent. In particular, discourses on HIV and AIDS can be linked to those concerning the risks of sexually transmitted infections, which were established during the colonial period as colonisers worried about the risks posed to White Europeans by infections such as syphilis, supposedly spread by colonised populations. This led to policies which as we argued previously with relation to sex work, criminalised and stigmatised African sexualities in an attempt to mitigate the "risk" to European populations whilst neglecting the health needs and rights of Africans themselves.

Following these colonial tropes of the need to control "risk", we can also highlight the ways in which the bio-medicalisation of the global HIV response and the framing of HIV infection as a global "risk", has frequently led to ignoring of the wider geopolitical contexts of this response, and notably the anchoring of much of the dominant discourses and policies within colonial and racist stereotypes concerning African sexual behaviour (e.g. frequency of multiple sexual partners), and implying that African countries do not have either the requisite government structures, nor adequate scientific knowledge, to be able to manage this epidemic without the intervention of countries from the Global North, and International Organisations.

The crudest or most basic of these discourses come back to the stereotypes of Africa as the "Dark Continent" (Jarosz, 1992), describing an African sexuality 'shorn of its political, economic and social context, and instead infused with moralising about unfettered African activity' (Jones, 2004, p. 192), resulting, as Flint and Hewitt argue, in the further entrenchment and othering of Africa as a "sick continent". Indeed, as they go on to argue, whilst discourses on HIV in other areas such as Asia might also have racist/colonial framings, 'where sub-Saharan HIV/AIDS (sic) has been concerned, the added element of sexual (and, significantly, heterosexual) transmission tapped into nineteenth-century colonial fixations in which degrees of "virtue" were linked to racial hierarchies' (Flint & Hewitt, 2015, p. 295). Further, these discourses also continue the colonial stereotypes of Africa as a continent in need of "governance", both in terms of moral governance of sexual behaviour and economic and political governance of health policies. The stereotype of morally promiscuous and "risky" sexual behaviour amongst Africans is thus perpetuated, leading to a focus in HIV and AIDS policies on stopping these "risky" behaviours and neglect of the wider socio-economic and political structures underlying the pandemic. As Danil (2021, p. 381) argues, 'A major reason for failures in the battle against HIV/AIDS (sic) in countries in sub-Saharan Africa has been argued to be the excessive focus placed on the notion that the problem stems from a culture of sexual promiscuity, moral shortcomings, and ignorance among Africans'.

This colonialist approach to HIV and AIDS, which sees the Global North as the repository of knowledge on how to "manage" the disease and positions the African continent as the site of "risk", is also linked to what has been called the securitisation of HIV and AIDS (O'Manique, 2005), where the pandemic was identified as an issue of national and international security. In 2000, the UN Security Council held the first session on HIV and AIDS, at which the then US Vice President, Al Gore, stated clearly:

> AIDS is not just a humanitarian crisis. It is a security crisis – because it threatens not just individual citizens, but the very institutions that define

and defend the character of a society. This disease weakens workforces and saps economic strength. AIDS strikes at teachers, and denies education to their students. It strikes at the military, and subverts the forces of order and peacekeeping.[4]

The securitisation of HIV and AIDS thus led to the understanding that the disease could be as much of a threat to national security and the integrity of state institutions as the military capabilities of other states (Elbe, 2011). On one hand, this could be seen to have positive impacts in placing HIV and AIDS high on the international agenda and leading to support for more investment and funding. However, this might have come at the price of handing over power to big international institutions, at the expense of local knowledge and socially rooted responses. As Elbe (2005) argues, the securitisation of HIV and AIDS has been responsible for the development of a global biopolitical economy of power dominated by the United States and other Western democracies through international multilateral organisations. In addition, it arguably came at the price of serious investment in HIV prevention. Elbe (2011, pp. 848–849) discusses the impacts of "securitisation" of health or "health security", which he asserts 'encourages the medicalisation of insecurity…(which includes) sustained attempts to secure populations through recourse to a growing array of pharmacological interventions'. As Conrad (1992, p. 211) explains, 'Medicalization (sic) consists of defining a problem in medical terms, using medical language to describe a problem, adopting a medical framework to understand a problem, or using a medical intervention to "treat" it'. This has led to the 'increased development, stockpiling and deployment of new medical countermeasures' (Elbe, 2011, p. 849) where the "solution" is on treatment rather than on the prevention of underlying structural inequalities, which render some more vulnerable than others.

## Treatment Over Prevention

Despite early and repeated calls around the importance of social change as the fundamental basis for prevention, biomedical interventions, initially to treat AIDS and more recently as a form of HIV prevention, have continued to dominate the HIV and AIDS response. And while the US President's Emergency Plan for AIDS Relief (PEPFAR) programme has indisputably been one of the most successful and largest funding initiatives to provide access to much-needed ART, it has also been a vehicle imbued with ideology around morality and sexual behaviour. In our earlier chapter, we drew attention to the prohibitions around including sex workers in care in the early roll out of the programme. These early years of the programme also saw the endorsement of non-evidence-based approaches, in particular the "abstain, be faithful and condomise" (popularly known as the "ABC") approach to prevention, which simplistically assumed capacity for unconstrained individual agency to actually achieve this. In fact, a third of PEPFAR's prevention funds were initially allocated to abstinence before marriage programmes (The Lancet Hiv, 2022). This context and framing have influenced the development of policies around HIV that have a narrow focus on addressing individual behaviour. These policies and programmes overlook structural drivers of disease and fail to grasp larger political, economic, and social factors (Danil, 2021; Hickel, 2012). In his analysis of donor prioritisations and channelling of bilateral funding for HIV, Jones shows that both NORAD and DFID, which nominally ground their approaches in human rights, in fact, prioritised funding for programmes targeting behavioural change and individual responsibility (Jones, 2011). This individual "behaviour change" approach is itself embedded in an idea of "risk", using epidemiological data to try and define the most "at risk" individuals or groups of individuals. Even when structural drivers started to be taken into consideration, this was within a public health framing with a focus on how structures and contexts influence individual risks and disease outcomes rather than looking at how structures of inequality distribute vulnerability and resilience unevenly across populations (O'Laughlin, 2015). As O'Laughlin (2015) maintains, the "social drivers" approach attempts to create models linking social variables such as gender, age, and class to individual behaviours and thus to individual health outcomes. The focus on individual-level behaviour persists with an emphasis that even though they may find themselves in positions of vulnerability because of social factors, individuals are still responsible for managing their own "risk" – also locating the idea of resilience as an individual capacity. As Anderson (2015, p. 21) explains, 'the invisibility and uncertainty of the risk posed by HIV has been confronted by medical science and clinical risk assessment, with an emphasis on the responsibilities of individuals for managing risk to their own bodies and selves'.

Another mechanism that has impacted the leverage of the United States in terms of donor assistance is the Mexico City Policy (or more commonly known as the "Global Gag Rule"), reinstated under successive Republican administrations and greatly expanded during the 2017–2021 term of then President Trump. The Global Gag Rule disqualifies foreign non-governmental organisations from eligibility for US Family Planning assistance if they use their own non-US funds to provide abortion services, counselling, or referrals or to advocate for the liberalising of abortion laws in their own country (Barot & Cohen, 2015). The expanded scope of the Mexico City Policy extends beyond US global family planning assistance to include almost all of US Global Health Assistance (called "Protecting Lives in Global Health Assistance"). Put into perspective, the United States has historically been the largest single donor of international population assistance and the largest donor for family planning and reproductive health (FP/RH) assistance in sub-Saharan Africa (Kates et al., 2018). During periods of policy enforcement, contraceptive and family planning services have been disrupted when NGOs were forced to cease their outreach activities, were faced with the closure of well-established clinics, and/or lost access to US-donated contraceptive commodities, thereby reducing the availability of contraceptives for women who require them (Barot & Cohen, 2015; Crane & Dusenberry, 2004; Jones, 2011). Several studies investigating the impact of the gag rule on abortion found that abortion rates increased in Africa during the periods that the gag rule was enforced (Bendavid et al., 2011; Jones, 2011). Indeed, the influence of donors on health priorities should not be underestimated. Shiffman and Smith (2007) conducted an illuminating analysis regarding factors that shaped political priority for the Global Safe Motherhood Initiative that was launched in 1987 to reduce maternal mortality but which two decades later failed to attract the necessary political support. Interestingly, concern around the US administration's conservatism regarding reproductive issues led to the Safe Motherhood Initiative being named as such because it was thought 'unlikely to incite active opposition from the administration' (p. 1375). The political consequences of a "motherhood" framing meant that the initiative received little attention from two key influencers – senior decision-makers and women's groups. Germane to our own analysis, those who were primarily affected – women in developing countries with little education and economic means – do not have much political power and are hampered in their actions by gender inequalities. They also lacked a recognised leader to champion on their behalf (Shiffman & Smith, 2007).

## What Does HIV Have to Do with SRHR?

As argued above, a rather narrow focus on HIV and AIDS can be seen to have led to neglect of wider SRHR issues, despite the inherent logic to pursue the interconnection between the two in policy and programming. While this line of reasoning received traction from the early 2000s onwards, the most notable advances have since been made in the integration of HIV counselling, testing and treatment services, and antenatal and postnatal services. Other linkages, including the promotion of condoms as a multi-purpose prevention tool, have been (much) less pursued at the service level due to the continuation of siloed sectors and funding for HIV and SRH (Kangudie et al., 2019; Warren et al., 2017). In terms of maternal and child health, tremendous successes have been seen in eliminating mother-to-child transmission of HIV (EMTCT) in sub-Saharan Africa, although there is indication that the early gains in averting HIV to newborns are slowly eroding (Poku et al., 2023). This is in part due to the long-standing neglect of the first and second pillars of EMTCT: the primary prevention of HIV among women of childbearing age and preventing unintended pregnancy amongst women living with HIV. With women seroconverting during pregnancy before being exposed to the EMTCT intervention, the risk of the foetus acquiring HIV in utero is extremely high. More recently, in SSA, there has been a push for treatment as prevention in the form of pre-exposure prophylaxis (PrEP) with sex workers, classed as "key populations", being initially targeted. Current formulations of PrEP provide no protection against STIs and pregnancy, although expanding these protections is in the research and development pipeline. While there is a fundamentally dynamic relationship between vulnerability to HIV acquisition and unintended pregnancy, this is not often seen to be acknowledged by the HIV community, which has tended to focus on HIV-related technologies in isolation from broader SRH needs. On a more obvious level, unprotected sex can lead to HIV acquisition, unintended pregnancy (assuming no contraceptive use), and a host of STIs, including HPV, which in turn heightens the biological risk of cervical cancer. However, pregnancy, in and of itself, may also increase susceptibility to HIV (Drake et al., 2014). On a more hidden level are the commonalities and unique interactions of determinants which may facilitate the relationship between unintended pregnancies and HIV incidence. It is no coincidence that countries with high rates of HIV also report low rates of contraceptive use, high rates of unmet need for contraception, and high rates of unintended pregnancy (Haddad et al., 2015; Hubacher et al., 2008). Yet, combination prevention[5] for adolescent girls and women consisting of integrated HIV, STI, and contraceptive services, recommended by the World Health Organisation as a priority action in countries with very high HIV prevalence and incidence rates, is rarely provided (WHO, 2020). In our Zimbabwe research, many young women did not cease selling sex while pregnant, with a number continuing to actively engage in sexual exchanges with different men until late in their third trimester of pregnancy, stopping selling sex briefly to give birth to their child, and returning within weeks of birth to selling sex. Research in other contexts has reported similar findings (Yam et al., 2017, Feldblum et al., 2007).

Given all of these linkages between HIV and SRHR, it is important to recognise that many key SRHR issues are still marginalised, impacting severely on women's health and rights. In the rest of the chapter, we go on to look at some of the key issues in SRHR in Southern Africa, showing, with examples from our research, that for young women, the main challenge is frequently not HIV.

## Early and Unintended Pregnancy

Almost half of all pregnancies worldwide are unintended (Bearak et al., 2020). Unintended pregnancies result in poor maternal and child health outcomes and are an indicator of 'global economic inequalities that influence people's ability to access sexual and reproductive health services' (Bearak et al., 2020, p. 1159). Compared to other regions, in 2023 the adolescent birth rate in sub-Saharan Africa remained amongst the highest in the world and particularly so for younger adolescent girls (10–14 years of age).[6] Adolescent girls disproportionately experience unintended pregnancies which often end in unsafe abortions (Sully et al., 2020). Not only is adolescent pregnancy a major contributor to adolescent maternal mortality and morbidity, it also disrupts childhood and schooling trajectories and perpetuates intergenerational cycles of ill-health and poverty (Nkwemu et al., 2019; UNESCO, 2017).

In the Southern African region, weak health systems and economic inequality have major impacts on young women's ability to access contraception. Stock outs, limited method mix, and provider-related barriers mean that services may be available in principle but not in practice, and many young women may have no alternative but to purchase contraception. However, as our research highlighted, the costs of these were often out of reach for the poorest and youngest women.

In Madagascar, young women explained that the constant shortage of contraceptive methods in public healthcare facilities meant that healthcare providers would push up prices for them. As one woman shared:

> Contraceptive injections should cost 500 ariary, but now they say there is a shortage and so they make you pay 3000 ariary. Girls went to the health centre to try and get the injection, but they only had 500 ariary, so they were turned away.
>
> *(20-year-old woman, Madagascar)*

As a result, many young women preferred to buy unregulated and/or expired contraceptives from black market providers in the streets, or else they would resort to traditional and less effective methods such as the rhythm method. Similar issues were found in Zimbabwe. One young woman explained to us:

> These days morning after pills are expensive, $15 bond, so if you get pregnant you abort.
>
> *(19-year-old woman, Zimbabwe)*

### *Impacts of Unintended Pregnancy*

Our research showed the importance of addressing the issue of early and unintended pregnancies amongst young women and, frequently, the lack of resources allocated to tackling this issue and supporting young women's rights. Again, intersecting inequalities create differing situations of vulnerability around pregnancy with the youngest girls and women most negatively affected. Research in Zambia highlights that high fertility also has important psychological, social, and economic consequences for adolescent girls' well-being, with pregnant girls being removed from or dropping out of school, facing violence or rejection from family members, as well as high levels of community censure (Zulu et al., 2024). The consequences of early and unintended pregnancy also negatively impact young women's mental health and well-being. Having child dependents greatly increases SRH vulnerability for young women in ways that are not experienced by young men. In Zambia, young girls who were able to return to school after the birth of their child struggled to catch up academically with their peers and faced a number of barriers in continuing school due to their altered life situation and the increased financial burden of having a child dependent (Zulu et al., 2024). More generally, research has shown that young women with no or low education and located in the lowest wealth quintile are disproportionately burdened with early childbearing (Bearak et al., 2020; Chung et al., 2018), with wide regional differences (Santhya & Jejeebhoy, 2015). Wealth inequalities are also known to affect access to safe abortion care, with women who are poorer and of lower socioeconomic class disproportionately disadvantaged (Chae et al., 2017; Zafar et al., 2018).

In our Zimbabwe research, 151 out of the 190 young women aged 16–24 years who participated in our FGDs indicated they had ever been pregnant; the mean age at first birth was 16.7 years (Chareka et al., 2021). In Madagascar, where according to available population-level data, 34.7% of young women between the ages of 15 and 19 have already had a child (Ravaoarisoa et al., 2020), the young women we spoke to talked about their fear of unintended pregnancy, which would be a "catastrophe" for them, leading to school drop out, economic precarity, and possible rejection by their partners and families (Freedman et al., 2020).

> It's true! If you become pregnant your future is ruined because you can't carry on with your studies, you won't be able to get a job.
>
> *(23-year-old woman, Madagascar)*

Often young people talked about the fact that if a young woman became pregnant, her partner would simply "run away":

> When girls get pregnant at 12 or 13, the father of the child might agree to pay some money, but generally they just run away. The majority of boys just run away.
>
> *(21-year-old woman, Madagascar)*

This finding that men frequently abandon their partner when she becomes pregnant was common across the study countries, relating to dominant gender norms around men's lack of accountability for parenthood. This may lead to a deepening of economic insecurity, which can push women into engaging in sexual-economic exchange (see Chapter 3). Indeed, across the region, the evidence suggests that child dependents in the absence of paternal support are key reasons for women to begin selling sex as a way to feed their children (Willis et al., 2016, Beckham et al, 2015, Gysels, Pool, & Nnalusiba, 2002, Agha & Chulu Nchima 2004).

In recognition of these challenges, there has been a global push to lower the age of consent for access to contraception to below 18 years (without requiring parental or spousal consent, as is still the case in many countries in the SSA). And while a number of countries in the Southern African region have successfully reduced the age, allowing women as young as 16 years old to be allowed to access contraception, young age still means women face numerous barriers at the point of service delivery. In Madagascar, for example, we found that despite the legal age of consent for access to contraception being lowered to 16, many service providers were still unaware of the reform and continued to ask young women to provide parental consent before accessing contraception (Freedman et al., 2020).

In Zimbabwe, young women talked about the difficulties of accessing contraception if they were considered "too young": 'Our age is the main barrier; they consider us too young to utilise the services' (19-year-old woman, Zimbabwe). At the time of the research, this young woman was financially supporting five dependents. She told us she first started selling sex at 16 years of age and had been pregnant three times. She had self-induced an abortion for each of these pregnancies.

In addition to young age being a barrier to accessing contraceptives, women's marital status and whether or not they have previously had children are also considered as part of their "eligibility" to access contraception from health service providers. Young women frequently told us that if they had not yet had a child, the clinic nurses frequently refused to provide them with contraception until they had had at least one child. One young woman in Zimbabwe explained:

> No it's not easy (to access contraception) because the (nurses) don't accept to give contraceptives to people without kids. They say you can become infertile and it affects you in the future. You need to tell them that you have a child (in order to obtain contraception).
>
> *(18-year-old woman, Zimbabwe)*

These myths about the use of contraception negatively impacting future fertility were widespread across all of the study countries, where, as we have noted, there is a gendered norm around the importance of fertility for young women. The above-quoted young woman was 15 years of age at her sexual debut. She had been pregnant twice before the age of 18 years with her first pregnancy, and the birth of her child was at 15 years of age. She had self-induced an abortion with her second pregnancy. At the time of the interview, she was supporting a household of four dependents.

A peer educator in another large city of Zimbabwe confirmed these accounts, highlighting that pregnancy was a precondition for access to contraception:

'Services such as family planning, they will never get those from the council clinic as long as they do not have a child. They can only get such service from the clinic if they get pregnant'. This demonstrates how young age, overlapping with legal, economic, and social insecurities, differentially shapes vulnerability for some young women. As we discussed in Chapter 3, for many young women we spoke to, pregnancy served as a catalyst for entry into sexual-economic exchanges and sex as a way to provide for a child (and other household dependents). Importantly, our research also highlights the strong role the community (including parents) can play in contributing to young women's vulnerable situations; this includes both the encouragement of young girls having children at an early age to demonstrate their fertility (Freedman et al., 2020), entering relationships characterised by sexual economic exchange, and participation in these relationships by male members of the same community (Zulu et al., 2024). Insights such as these strongly challenge the view of focusing on individual behaviours and understandings around risk.

Our previous research in South Africa found that unintended pregnancy could have a destabilising effect on women's social support structures through increased conflict in family and partner relationships due to economic insecurities (Lewinsohn et al., 2018). The lack of familial support networks was particularly marked in relation to pregnancy and childcare amongst young refugee women in our South African research (Crankshaw et al., 2023). Young women pointed to these support networks as what they perceived to be a key difference between their situation and that of their South African peers, who are more likely to have their mothers or grandmothers assist with child care. As with our other study countries, a number of young women spoke about being deserted by the father of the child, thus leaving young women refugees with little support in the context of deepened levels of economic insecurity:

> He went there to the Eastern Cape and he left me here with the pregnancy. He went for like 6 months and he never came back. He was talking to me but he never came back, he never sent anything and I said, 'Haibo, I can't be sitting by myself in this house!' He was paying the rent for the house when he was there and when he stopped paying, I said, 'Eish, I can't survive!'
>
> *(23-year-old Congolese woman, South Africa)*

## Access to Safe Abortion

In response to an unwanted pregnancy, women may choose to exercise their reproductive right to terminate the pregnancy. However, a combination of restrictive abortion laws, abortion stigma, and/or procedural hurdles at the service level seriously constrain women's access to a safe abortion on the continent (Berer, 2017; Blystad et al., 2019). Legally restricting abortion does not stop abortions from occurring; it just makes them less safe since they are carried out in a clandestine manner and often through informal providers who may use unsafe methods. This is particularly the case for the youngest and poorest, with those with the most resources being able to access safe abortion care at a cost. Restricted options also create space for exploitation by unscrupulous providers of women desperate to end an unwanted pregnancy. In countries with very restrictive abortion laws and policies, the cost of accessing abortion becomes prohibitively high for many women.

> … if they prescribe medication for you, the medication is sold in USD and we charge our clients in Bond (Zimbabwean currency of lower value). So where are we supposed to get the USD? You will be lucky to get USD from a client, it's like a shooting star to get a client who pays in USD.
>
> *(18-year-old woman, Zimbabwe)*

In Madagascar, for example, the price of over-the-counter medical abortion pills was found to be extremely high relative to the minimum wage in the country (Pourette et al., 2018).

In high-income countries where abortion is broadly legal, it has been found that the abortion rate and proportion of unintended pregnancies ending in abortion are the lowest, as is the rate of unintended pregnancy (Bearak et al., 2020), underlining the fact of better overall SRHR outcomes in contexts where reproductive rights are supported. Conversely, the proportion of unintended pregnancies ending in abortion has been found to be the highest in countries where abortion is legally restricted (Bearak et al., 2020).

Our and other research suggests that abortions are common amongst young women in the region. In Madagascar, for example, nearly 60% of young women interviewed who had an unintended pregnancy had resorted to abortion (Freedman et al., 2020). In Zimbabwe, nearly one-third (30%) of young women aged 16–24 years reported ever having an abortion, of these 23% reporting abortion-related complications (Chareka et al., 2021). Eighteen (41%) of the Zimbabwean participants who had undergone an abortion had done so more than once (Ibid). These abortions occur despite the restrictive legal context, which we discussed in Chapter 1.

In all countries in which we carried out our research, young women frequently had recourse to "traditional" methods to terminate unwanted pregnancies. In our research in Madagascar, where the illegality of abortion makes it nearly impossible to access medical abortion, many young women talked about using herbs or herbal drinks to try and terminate unwanted pregnancies:

> You are still a schoolgirl and you already have a boyfriend, so you feel like you have to have sex with him. And then you get pregnant. You're scared of

> your parents so you ask your schoolfriends what to do. And they advise you to drink bitter herbal drinks to provoke an abortion. There are girls who die because there are remains of the pregnancy in their uterus.
>
> *(20-year-old woman, Madagascar)*

Others talked about going to visit “matrones”, women who would massage their stomachs to try and provoke an abortion, or taking large doses of medication purchased in pharmacies. Some even suggested introducing soap into the vagina, jumping up and down repeatedly, or riding a bicycle for a long time as methods to try and induce abortion (Freedman et al., 2020).

In Zimbabwe, there was significant fear amongst younger women that they would face punitive consequences if their abortion was discovered by health care providers:

> We make sure we do everything at home because the older (sex workers) told us that if you just get to the clinic they will report you to the police. We fear failure to answer questions at the clinic so we don’t go to the clinic.
>
> *(18-year-old woman, Zimbabwe)*

Uncertainties around or knowledge of the legal context around the termination of pregnancies in Zimbabwe and Zambia were key determinants underlying the clandestine nature of abortions. This lack of knowledge about abortion law is echoed in the existing literature in the region (Assifi et al., 2016; Cresswell et al., 2016; Fetters et al., 2017; Mekuria et al., 2020; Sheehy et al., 2021). And while age and socioeconomic concerns were key in decision-making around abortions, socioeconomic status also determined whether a young girl could access quality care at a private provider or whether a traditional healer or older woman in the community conducted the procedure, often using unsafe methods (Chareka et al., 2021). In Zimbabwe, youth, cost, and a lack of referral networks contributed towards unsafe abortions, even when safe abortion services (through private facilities) are available. Socio-economic status was also a major factor in the ability to access abortion in Madagascar, as young women who have enough money are able to pay doctors who will carry out abortions clandestinely, even though this is illegal. We were told in Zambia that ‘those with money ... can do things in secrecy’ (Zulu et al., 2024, page 9), meaning that should a girl and/or family have the ability to afford a safe abortion at a private clinic, they were also assured of the confidentiality that comes with private care. In Madagascar, women who have the necessary economic resources often travel to neighbouring countries, such as Mauritius, to access an abortion.

In many cases, there is also shame and stigma attached to seeking an abortion, and this is worsened in situations where abortion is criminalised. When young women are known to have undergone an abortion, this can lead to a loss of emotional and economic support from family or a partner (Chemlal & Russo, 2019) or exclusion from family and community. Again, women with better socio-economic resources are far less exposed to the risk of complications arising from unsafe methods, which would reveal that they had undergone an abortion in the first place, and so suffer less from this type of stigma. Lastly, girls from wealthier families are more able to conceal their pregnancies until they could obtain an abortion since they mixed less within the community and, as such, were not subjected to community scrutiny in ways that young girls from poor families are (Zulu et al., 2024).

Even in countries where abortions are allowed on specific grounds, the procedural hurdles required to actually obtain the service often mean that public sector care is, in reality, not an option. As part of monitoring the SDG goal of ensuring universal SRHR, the United Nations developed indicator 5.6.2, which provides an assessment of the legal environment related to SRHR. Only 8% of the 87 countries that reported on the abortion indicator indicated that they had the full set of laws and regulations in place enabling access to abortion. On the other hand, 99% of the 107 countries that provided information indicated that they had the required laws and regulations in place for post-abortion care (PAC) (UNFPA 2021). Our research confirmed the paradox of the widespread availability of PAC while women are simultaneously denied the right to a legal and safe abortion. In these contexts, PAC is in place as an emergency intervention to deal with the complications arising from unsafe abortions, rather than part of a comprehensive package of SRH care that is intended to be available (WHO, 2022). Even where abortions were legally permitted on a number of grounds, young women did not generally access this care for fear of being arrested, for reasons of confidentiality, or for a lack of knowledge of the conditions under which an abortion may be legally allowed. On the other hand, we found that PAC services are widely known about and, depending on the context, are accessed out of medical necessity. However, accessing PAC also created a space for young women to be chastised and frequently treated cruelly by health care professionals.

> After some examinations at the hospital, they discovered I had aborted; they did not give any injection to numb the pain while cleaning me; they cleaned me just like that …and said I should never abort again.
>
> *(18-year-old woman, Zambia)*

The increasingly restrictive context around abortion and the impacts of global anti-gender campaigns have been felt in the region, with not only barriers to the liberalisation of abortion laws but also a deeper criminalisation of abortion in some countries. In Madagascar, for example, since a proposed reform of the abortion law to allow therapeutic abortion was rejected in 2017, surveillance of doctors practicing abortions in secret has increased, and many have stopped offering this service as a consequence and for fear of being condemned to prison if they are discovered. A second attempt to debate the issue in parliament in 2021 was cut short when a newly proposed bill was withdrawn without discussion. The space for women to exercise their reproductive rights is also narrowing in other countries like Zambia, with providers fearing punitive consequences if found to be providing abortion, on the one hand, and increased political control over the contents of sexuality education as a preventive tool on the other hand (Zulu & Haaland, 2019).

## Conclusions

"But what about the men?" This question is repeatedly asked when we present our research on SRHR in various fora, both academic and non-academic. In all of our research on SRHR, we have noticed that whilst there may be, in some cases, lip service paid to women's rights and the importance of SRHR, in fact, these are a range of health issues which continue to be marginalised. Early and unintended pregnancy and access to contraception, for example, are seen as women's issues and thus arguably less important as national or global health issues. The only exception is that of HIV and AIDS, which, as we have argued in this chapter, have been represented and understood as a threat to national and international health "security" in such a way as to attract important international attention and donor funding. High levels of unintended pregnancies are not seen as "threats" in the same way as HIV and AIDS prevalence. Whilst women have in theory been "included" within the HIV and AIDS response, as we have shown, this inclusion remains very much at the level of community-based responses, with major decision-making powers and funding still mainly in male hands. The failure to take other SRHR issues seriously and to really consider women's needs and women's rights has, we would argue, made it easier for the current anti-gender movements to mobilise against rights such as access to safe abortion by opening up a space where these rights have already been marginalised and to categorically refute the link between structural poverty, gender inequalities, and poor SRHR. And paradoxically, whilst the response to HIV and AIDS can be seen to be framed in very colonialist terms with its understandings of women's sexualities as a health "risk" that needs to be managed, the anti-gender movements in Southern Africa have managed to subvert this framing by claiming that their opposition to abortion rights should be understood as a resistance to the imposition of Western or colonial values in the region. Despite the fact that most Southern African countries still bear the legacy of restrictive colonial-era legislation around termination of pregnancy, one of the arguments employed by opponents of the liberalisation of existing abortion laws explicitly links the "liberalisation agenda" with colonialism, arguing that abortion is a Western agenda consisting of 'westerners imposing cultural and linguistic features on African life' (Chisweshe & Macleod, 2018, p. 51).

What is overlooked and neglected in all of this is the fact that women are frequently found in the most vulnerable health situations, made vulnerable by an intersecting matrices of inequalities, within which gender inequality continues to be central. And when these gender inequalities and women's continuing vulnerability are questioned, the response is still too often: "but what about the men?"

## Notes

1 https://www.unaids.org/en/topic/key-populations
2 https://www.theglobalfund.org/en/key-populations/
3 Defined by UNAIDS as "sex workers and their clients, gay men and other men who have sex with men, people who inject drugs, transgender people".
4 Vice President Al Gore, Statement in the Security Council on AIDS in Africa January 10, 2000, available at: http://www.un.int/usa/00_002.htm
5 Combination prevention is also one of the five pillars in the HIV Prevention 2025 Roadmap and includes a span of services, notably comprehensive sexuality education, HIV and SRH services (including male and female condoms and other contraceptive tools), ART-based prevention and harm reduction for women who use drugs, and interventions to change harmful gender norms, end gender-based discrimination, inequalities and violence, improve social protection and support economic empowerment. (UNAIDS, 2022)
6 https://www.who.int/news-room/fact-sheets/detail/adolescent-pregnancy

## References

Agha, S. & Chulu Nchima, M. (2004). Life-circumstances, working conditions and HIV risk among street and nightclub-based sex workers in Lusaka, Zambia. *Culture, Health & Sexuality*, *6*(4), 283–299.

Anderson, E. L. (2015). *Gender, HIV and risk.* Palgrave Macmillan.

Assifi, A. R., Berger, B., Tunçalp, Ö, Khosla, R., & Ganatra, B. (2016). Women's awareness and knowledge of abortion laws: A systematic review. *PloS One*, *11*(3), e0152224.

Barot, S., & Cohen, S. A. (2015). The global gag rule and fights over funding UNFPA: The issues that Won't go away. *Guttmacher Policy Review*, *18*(2), 27–33.

Bearak, J., Popinchalk, A., Ganatra, B., Moller, A. B., Tunçalp, Ö, Beavin, C., Kwok, L., & Alkema, L. (2020). Unintended pregnancy and abortion by income, region, and the legal status of abortion: Estimates from a comprehensive model for 1990–2019. *The Lancet Global Health*, *8*(9), e1152–e1161.

Beckham, S. W., Shembilu, C. R., Winch, P. J., Beyrer, C., & Kerrigan, D. L. J. C. (2015). 'If you have children, you have responsibilities': Motherhood, sex work and HIV in Southern Tanzania. *Health & Sexuality*, *17*(2), 165–179.

Bendavid, E., Avila, P., & Miller, G. (2011). United States aid policy and induced abortion in sub-Saharan Africa. *Bulletin of the World Health Organisation*, *89*, 873–880c.

Berer, M. (2017). Abortion law and policy around the world: In search of decriminalization. *Health and Human Rights*, *19*(1), 13.

Blystad, A., Haukanes, H., Tadele, G., Haaland, M. E., Sambaiga, R., Zulu, J. M., & Moland, K. M. (2019). The access paradox: Abortion law, policy and practice in Ethiopia, Tanzania and Zambia. *International Journal for Equity in Health*, *18*, 1–15.

Chae, S., Desai, S., Crowell, M., & Sedgh, G. (2017). Reasons why women have induced abortions: A synthesis of findings from 14 countries. *Contraception*, *96*(4), 233–241.

Chareka, S., Crankshaw, T. L., & Zambezi, P. (2021). Economic and social dimensions influencing safety of induced abortions amongst young women who sell sex in Zimbabwe. *Sexual and Reproductive Health Matters*, *29*(1), 121–132.

Chemlal, S., Russo, G. (2019). Why do they take the risk? A systematic review of the qualitative literature on informal sector abortions in settings where abortion is legal. *BMC Women's Health*, *19*, 1–11.

Chiweshe, M., & Macleod, C. (2018). Cultural de-colonization versus liberal approaches to abortion in Africa: The politics of representation and voice. *African Journal of Reproductive Health*, *22*(2), 49–59.

Chung, H. W., Kim, E. M., & Lee, J. E. (2018). Comprehensive understanding of risk and protective factors related to adolescent pregnancy in low-and middle-income countries: A systematic review. *Journal of Adolescence*, *69*, 180–188.

Conrad, P. (1992). Medicalization and social control. *Annual Review of Sociology*, *18*(1), 209–232.

Crane, B. B., & Dusenberry, J. (2004). Power and politics in international funding for reproductive health: The US global gag rule. *Reproductive Health Matters*, *12*(24), 128–137.

Crankshaw, T. L., Muparamoto, N., Chareka, S., & Ngwenya, P. (2023). Intersectional vulnerabilities and differential impacts of COVID-19 responses on young people who sell sex in Zimbabwe. *Culture, Health & Sexuality*, *25*(7), 818–832.

Cresswell, J. A., Schroeder, R., Dennis, M., Owolabi, O., Vwalika, B., Musheke, M., Campbell, O., & Filippi, V. (2016). Women's knowledge and attitudes surrounding abortion in Zambia: A cross-sectional survey across three provinces. *BMJ Open*, *6*(3), e010076.

Danil, L. R. (2021). Queerphobic immunopolitics in the case of HIV/AIDS: Political economy, the dark legacy of British colonialism, and queerphobia in Sub-Saharan Africa. *Sexuality & Culture*, *25*(2), 377–395.

Drake, A. L., Wagner, A., Richardson, B., & John-Stewart, G. (2014). Incident HIV during pregnancy and postpartum and risk of mother-to-child HIV transmission: A systematic review and meta-analysis. *PLoS Medicine*, *11*(2), e1001608.

Elbe, S. (2005). AIDS, security, biopolitics. *International Relations*, *19*(4), 403–419.

Elbe, S. (2011). Pandemics on the radar screen: Health security, infectious disease and the medicalisation of insecurity. *Political Studies*, *59*(4), 848–866.

Feldblum, P. J., Nasution, M. D., Hoke, T. H., et al. (2007). Pregnancy among sex workers participating in a condom intervention trial highlights the need for dual protection. *Contraception*, *76*(2), 105–110.

Fetters, T., Samandari, G., Djemo, P., Vwallika, B., & Mupeta, S. (2017). Moving from legality to reality: How medical abortion methods were introduced with implementation science in Zambia. *Reproductive Health*, *14*, 1–11.

Flint, A., & Hewitt, V. (2015). Colonial tropes and HIV/AIDS in Africa: Sex, disease and race. *Commonwealth & Comparative Politics*, *53*(3), 294–314.

Freedman, J., Rakatoarindrasata, M., & Randrianasolorivo, J. D. (2020). *Santé sexuelle et reproductive chez les jeunes 'populations clés' à Madagascar*. HEARD.

Gysels, M., Pool, R, & Nnalusiba, B. (2002). Women who sell sex in a Ugandan trading town: Life histories, survival strategies and risk. *Social Science & Medicine*, *54*(2), 179–192.

Haddad, L. B., Philpott-Jones, S., & Schonfeld, T. (2015). Contraception and prevention of HIV transmission: A potential conflict of public health principles. *Journal of Family Planning and Reproductive Health Care*, *41*(1), 20–23.

Harman, S. (2011). The dual feminisation of HIV/AIDS. *Globalizations*, *8*(2), 213–228.

Harrison, A., Short, S., & Tuoane, M. (2014). Re-focusing the gender lens: Caregiving women, family roles and HIV/AIDS vulnerability in Lesotho. *AIDS Behavior*, *18*(3), 595–604.

Heywood, M. (2020). The transformative power of civil society in South Africa: An activist's perspective on innovative forms of organizing and rights-based practices. *Globalizations*, *17*(2), 294–316.

Hickel, J. (2012). Neoliberal plague: The political economy of HIV transmission in Swaziland. *Journal of Southern African Studies*, *38*(3), 513–529.

Hosegood, V., Preston-Whyte, E., Busza, J., Moitse, S., & Timaeus, I. M. (2007). Revealing the full extent of households' experiences of HIV and AIDS in rural South Africa. *Social Science & Medicine*, *65*(6), 1249–59.

Hubacher, D., Mavranezouli, I., & McGinn, E. (2008). Unintended pregnancy in sub-Saharan Africa: Magnitude of the problem and potential role of contraceptive implants to alleviate it. *Contraception*, *78*(1), 73–78.

Iversen, J., Page, K., Madden, A., & Maher, L. (2015). HIV, HCV, and health-related harms among women who inject drugs: Implications for prevention and treatment. *Journal of Acquired Immune Deficiency Syndrome*, *69*(Suppl 2), S176–S181.

Jarosz, L. (1992). Constructing the dark continent: Metaphor as geographic representation of Africa. *Geografiska Annaler: Series B, Human Geography*, *74*(2), 105–115.

Jones, J. (2011). Ebola, emerging: The limitations of culturalist discourses in epidemiology. *The Columbia University Journal of Global Health*, *1*(1), 1–6.

Jones, P. S. (2004). When 'development' devastates: Donor discourses, access to HIV/AIDS treatment in Africa and rethinking the landscape of development. *Third World Quarterly*, *25*(2), 385–404.

Kangudie, D. M., Guidigbi, H., Mensah, S., Bala, A. A., & Delate, R. (2019). Effective integration of sexual reproductive health and HIV prevention, treatment, and care services across sub-Saharan Africa: Where is the evidence for program implementation? *Reproductive Health*, *16*(Suppl 1), 56.

Kates, J., Wexler, A., & Lief, E. (November 2018). Donor government funding for family planning in 2017. *The Kaiser Family Foundation*. https://www.google.com/url?sa=t&source=web&rct=j&opi=89978449&url=https://files.kff.org/attachment/Report-Donor-Government-Funding-for-Family-Planning-in-2017&ved=2ahUKEwjM9O-T96WHAxWzU0EAHaSnAHYQFnoECBEQAQ&usg=AOvVaw3g2Y9c3U4caTts_teO7jQL

Lewinsohn, R., Crankshaw, T., Tomlinson, M., Gibbs, A., Butler, L., & Smit, J. (2018). This baby came up and then he said, "I give up!": The interplay between unintended pregnancy, sexual partnership dynamics and social support and the impact on women's well-being in KwaZulu-Natal, South Africa. *Midwifery*, *62*, 29–35.

Mekuria, M., Daba, D., Girma, T., & Birhanu, A. (2020). Assessment of knowledge on abortion law and factors affecting it among regular undergraduate female students of Ambo University, Oromia Region, Ethiopia, 2018: a cross sectional study. Contraception and Reproductive Medicine, 5, 1–8.

Merson, M. H., O'Malley, J., Serwadda, D., & Apisuk, C. (2008). The history and challenge of HIV prevention. *The Lancet*, *372*(9637), 475–488.

Nkwemu, S., Jacobs, C. N., Mweemba, O., Sharma, A., & Zulu, J. M. (2019). "They say that I have lost my integrity by breaking my virginity": Experiences of teen school going mothers in two schools in Lusaka Zambia. *BMC Public Health*, *19*, 1–8.

O'Laughlin, B. (2015). Trapped in the prison of the proximate: Structural HIV/AIDS prevention in Southern Africa. *Review of African Political Economy*, *42*(145), 342–361.

O'Manique, C. (2005). The "securitisation" of HIV/AIDS in Sub-Saharan Africa: A critical feminist lens. *Policy and Society*, *24*(1), 24–47.

Parker, R. (2011). Grassroots activism, civil society mobilization, and the politics of the global HIV/AIDS epidemic. *The Brown Journal of World Affairs*, *17*(2), 21–37.

Poku, N. K., Strauss, M., Crankshaw, T. L., & Chareka, S. (2023). *Sexual and reproductive health and rights in Eastand Southern Africa*. Health Economics and HIV and AIDS Research Division, University of KwaZulu-Natal.

Pourette, D., Mattern, C., Ratovoson, R., Raharimalala, P. (2018). Complications with use of misoprostol for abortion in Madagascar: Between ease of access and lack of information. *Contraception*, *97*(2), 116–121.

Ramjee, G., & Daniels, B. (2013). Women and HIV in sub-Saharan Africa. *AIDS Research and Therapy*, *10*, 1–9.

Ravaoarisoa, L., Razafimahatratra, M. J. J., Rakotondratsara, M. A., Gaspard, N., Ratsimbazafy, M. R., Rafamantanantsoa, J. F., & Casey, S. E. (2020). Slowing progress: The US global Gag rule undermines access to contraception in Madagascar. *Sexual and Reproductive Health Matters*, *28*(3), 39–53.

Risher, K. A., Cori, A., Reniers, G., Marston, M., Calvert, C., Crampin, A., & Eaton, J. W. (2021). Age patterns of HIV incidence in eastern and southern Africa: A modelling analysis of observational population-based cohort studies. *The Lancet HIV*, *8*(7), e429–e439.

Santhya, K. G., & Jejeebhoy, S. J. (2015). Sexual and reproductive health and rights of adolescent girls: Evidence from low-and middle-income countries. *Global Public Health*, *10*(2), 189–221.

Sheehy, G., Dozier, J. L., Mickler, A. K., Yihdego, M., Karp, C., & Zimmerman, L. A. (2021). Regional and residential disparities in knowledge of abortion legality and availability of facility-based abortion services in Ethiopia. *Contraception: X*, *3*, 100066.

Shiffman, J., & Smith, S. (2007). Generation of political priority for global health initiatives: A framework and case study of maternal mortality. *The Lancet*, *370*(9595), 1370–1379.

Sully, E. A., Biddlecom, A., Darroch, J. E., Riley, T., Ashford, L. S., Lince-Deroche, N., & Murro, R. (2020). *Adding it up: Investing in sexual and reproductive health 2019*. Guttmacher Institute.

The Lancet Hiv. (2022). *PEPFAR looks to the future*. *Lancet HIV*, *9*(6), e367. doi: 10.1016/S2352-3018(22)00141-2.

UNAIDS. (2022). *HIV prevention 2025 roadmap. Getting on track to end AIDS as a public health threat by 2030*. UNAIDS.

UNAIDS, (2023). *Programme on HIV/AIDS. The path that ends AIDS. UNAIDS global AIDS update 2023*. UNAIDS.

UNESCO. (2017). *Early and unintended pregnancy and the education sector: Evidence review and recommendations*. UNESCO.

UNFPA. (2021). "My body is my own. Claiming the right to autonomy and self-determination". State of the world population 2021. Available: https://www.unfpa.org/publications/state-world-population-2021

Warren, C. E., Hopkins, J., Narasimhan, M., Collins, L., Askew, I., & Mayhew, S. H. (2017). Health systems and the SDGs: Lessons from a joint HIV and sexual and reproductive health and rights response. *Health Policy and Planning*, *32*(Suppl_4), iv102–iv107.

Watkins-Hayes, C. (2014). Intersectionality and the sociology of HIV/AIDS: Past, present, and future research directions. *Annual Review of Sociology*, *40*, 431–457.
Willis, B., Welch, K., & Onda, S. (2016). Health of female sex workers and their children: A call for action. *The Lancet Global Health*, *4*(7), e438–e439.
World Health Organisation. (2020). *Actions for improved clinical and prevention services and choices. Preventing HIV and other sexually transmitted infections among women and girls using contraceptive services in contexts with high HIV incidence.*
World Health Organisation (2022). *Abortion care guideline*.
Yam Eileen A., Aklilu Kidanu, Burnett-Zieman Brady, et al. (2017). Pregnancy experiences of female sex workers in Adama City, Ethiopia: Complexity of partner relationships and pregnancy intentions. *Studies in Family Planning*, *48*(2), 107–119.
Zafar, H., Ameer, H., Fiaz, R., Aleem, S., Abid, S., & Aleem, M. S. (2018). Low socioeconomic status leading to unsafe abortion-related complications: A third-world country dilemma. *Cureus*, *10*(10).
Zulu, J. M., & Haaland, M. E. (2019). Situating the Mexico City Policy: What shapes contraceptive access and abortion? *The Lancet Global Health*, *7*(8), e984–e985.
Zulu, J. Crankshaw, T.L, Ouedraogo, R., Juma, K., Aantjes, C.J. (2024). "The ones at the bottom of the food chain": structural drivers of unintended pregnancy and unsafe abortion amongst adolescent girls in Zambia. *Archives of Public Health 82*, 1–13.

# 5

# SEXUAL AND GENDER-BASED VIOLENCE

## The Most Pressing Challenge for SRHR?

### Introduction

Despite various international, regional, and national conventions and legal frameworks on the prevention and eradication of sexual and gender-based violence (SGBV)[1] and a range of programmes and activities which have been initiated by international and national organisations to combat violence, SGBV remains a massive problem globally (Hayes, 2007). Nearly one in three women (31%) worldwide have been subjected to physical and/or sexual violence from an intimate partner or sexual violence by a non-partner, or to both of these forms of violence at least once from the age of 15 years (WHO, 2021). Intimate partner violence (IPV) starts early in women's lives; almost one in four (24%) ever-partnered adolescent girls aged 15–19 years were estimated to have been subjected to such violence at least once in their lifetime (WHO 2021). Children growing up with violence are more likely to experience or perpetrate violence themselves in the future. There is a growing recognition that SGBV poses a significant obstacle and challenge to development, both because it is a direct infringement of women's human rights and because of its economic, social, and political costs (Hughes et al., 2016). There is also growing evidence of the wide-ranging short and long-term health consequences of SGBV. SGBV is a cause of mortality, but it is also associated with a range of other negative health outcomes, including physical injury, HIV and other sexually transmitted infections, unwanted pregnancy, or pregnancy complications, trauma, and mental health problems (Jewkes, 2002). However, as we will argue, the consequences of SGBV are not merely health related. Garcia-Moreno (2002) stresses the need to look beyond physical injury as a measure of SGBV because it does not provide

DOI: 10.4324/9781003414698-5

a broad enough framework to understand all of the forms and consequences of violence. Impacts on women's mental health, for example, may frequently be ignored if we look only at the physical effects of violence. And experiencing SGBV may negatively impact a whole range of other areas of life, such as education, employment, etc. There is a need to better understand the broad range of consequences of SGBV and of the interlinkages between them. And all of these multiple and long-term consequences have major costs at the individual level and at the level of families, communities, and societies as a whole, particularly as health, legal, and social services to help those who have experienced violence overcome the negative consequences of SGBV are not always available or accessible. The inaccessibility of health care for victims of SGBV also poses a problem of health equity, adding to the gendered inequalities in access to health care.

The probability of experiencing SGBV is not the same for all women, which is why it is important to adopt an intersectional approach to understand how and why women may be vulnerable to experiencing SGBV and how this situated intersectionality also impacts their ability to seek support if they do experience violence. Other factors such as age, social class and status, race and ethnicity, migration status, disability, sexual orientation, gender identity, for example, all influence women's vulnerability to and experience of violence. For example, the evidence suggests that the prevalence of both lifetime violence and violence experienced in the past 12 months amongst ever-married or partnered women was highest among least developed countries (37% and 22%, respectively) (WHO, 2021). Sub-Saharan Africa is amongst the regions with the highest prevalence rates of IPV over a lifetime (33%) and over the past 12 months (20%) (WHO, 2021). The Southern Africa region reflects similarly high rates of SGBV against women and girls; compared to the global average of 27%, country prevalence estimates of lifetime IPV amongst every married or partnered woman (15–49 years) in the following countries are: Zimbabwe (35%), Zambia (41%), South Africa (24%), and Mozambique (30%) (WHO, 2021). In Madagascar, 41% of ever partnered women have experienced at least one form of IPV (World Bank, 2023). Sexual violence in early adolescence (10–14 years) is high, with more than 20–40% of young girls who report sexual violence experiencing it before the age of 15 years in Zimbabwe, Zambia, and Mozambique, respectively (UNICEF, 2014).

## Understanding the Continuum(s) of Violence

In order to analyse and understand differential vulnerabilities to SGBV and also the varying consequences of SGBV depending on a person's intersectional location, we first need to arrive at a definition of what SGBV is, something which has not always been clear either in research or policy. The UN Declaration on the

Elimination of Violence Against Women (adopted on 20 December 1993, General Assembly resolution 48/104)[2] defines this violence as 'any act of gender-based violence that results in, or is likely to result in, physical, sexual or psychological harm or suffering to women, including threats of such acts, coercion or arbitrary deprivation of liberty, whether occurring in public or in private life' (p. 2). One definition that has been widely accepted in the humanitarian context is that SGBV is 'an umbrella term used to define any harmful act that is perpetrated against a person's will, and that is based on socially ascribed (gender) differences between males and females' (Inter-Agency Standing Committee, 2015, p. 5). This is commonly understood to include physical, emotional, sexual, and psychological acts, attempts, and threats. More recently, the understanding of SGBV has been extended to include other harmful practices such as female genital mutilation (FGM), child marriage, early childbearing and trafficking, and sexual violence as a weapon of war.

However, despite these definitions, one of the problems which emerges from a review of the academic and policy literature on SGBV is the lack of a clear definition of what constitutes this violence and where its limits are situated, despite various definitions in international conventions. For some, SGBV is synonymous with violence against women (Terry, 2007), whilst for others it is a much broader term which encompasses a wide range of different forms of gendered and sexualised violence against both women and girls and men and boys, as well as against persons of diverse sexual orientations, gender identities, and expressions (SOGIE) (Graaff, 2021; Read-Hamilton, 2014). Some have suggested that since gender relations permeate all social relationships, all violence is in fact gendered, and thus the use of the term "gender-based violence" is erroneous in which it suggests that 'forms of violence exist which are unrelated to processes of gender/sexual positioning and broader social gender inequalities' (Leach & Humphreys, 2007, p. 108). When the term gender-based violence was first employed, it was used to move beyond a simple differentiation between men and women based on biological sex and to denote the ways in which violence against women (or, in some cases, men) is based on gendered social norms and structures, and thus to link individual acts of violence to wider social constructions. This usage is important in reminding us of the origins and causes of gender-based violence and in moving away from individualistic explanations of such violence. By linking individual acts of violence to social norms, values, and structures, the issue of violence against women becomes politicised, suggesting that the means of prevention do not just lie in the treatment of individual cases and that wider social, political, and economic reforms are needed in order to prevent violence against women. However, it can be argued that over time, the usage of the concept of gender-based violence has become more vague and variable as it has expanded in an effort to include multiple different forms of violence, and that as this has happened, the important causal linkages to underlying structural gender inequalities have sometimes been lost, and thus it might be argued that a depoliticisation of the issues has taken place (Cornwall et al., 2007). In particular, a push to recognise gendered violence against men and boys, including rape and sexual violence against men in conflict, which is often underreported (Scully, 2009), and to include this in campaigns for the prevention and elimination of violence and treatment of survivors has widened into a more general imperative to "include men and boys" without any real definitions of what this "inclusion" actually means. In fact, some of this work may be counterproductive in 'framing violence in terms of culture and not politics, socialisation not oppression' (Greig, 2011, p. 225). Thus, the widening of the use of the concept of gender-based violence to include men, whilst welcome in theory, as a recognition that men can also be victims of forms of violence based on gendered norms and structures, has in practice sometimes led to an over-stretching of the category of gender-based violence, which has in turn depoliticised it. Moreover, "adding" men and boys into programmes or policies designed to address violence against women and girls does not consider the ways in which men themselves are gendered. Recognising that certain forms of masculinities may be linked to gendered violence and that these masculinities are damaging for both men and women is clearly valuable, but if these masculinities are located solely within male bodies, without linking them to political and economic structures and the violence of the state, then the relationships between individual violence and the violence of social structures are left unexplored (Greig, 2011).

To understand the ways in which gender-based violence impacts men, it is necessary to analyse the ways in which political, social, and economic structures of gender inequality affect men's lives in ways that are different from the impacts on women's lives (Ratele, 2014; Shefer et al., 2010). As Read-Hamilton (2014) argues, merely adding men and boys to strategies and policies aimed at the prevention of violence against women does not make sense from a theoretical or practical perspective, as it fails to acknowledge that the causes and consequences of sexualised and gendered violence against men and boys are not the same as those of violence against women. This blurring of the category of gender-based violence and a widening use of the term gender have resulted in a situation in which violence is often referred to as "gendered" without any real understanding or explanation of how or why it is gendered or what this really means (Scully, 2010). Assuming that all forms of violence against women are "gender-based" without analysing this violence in relation to specific theories and meanings of gender can be seen as a failure to analyse the "gender-violence nexus" in the light of all the theorisation of gender and gendered social relations and inequalities of power (Anderson, 2009).

Paying attention to violence against women does not mean ignoring the fact that men and boys can be victims of gendered forms of violence. It is a recognition that women and girls are the primary victims and that the gendered structures of inequality within which this violence is based (and which is in turn reinforced) are structures within which women are dominated within the varying hierarchies of power. In this sense, Jakobsen (2014) suggests the importance of seeing gender both as a practice and as the result of practice, whereby practices of gendering create and reinforce the gender norms and values upon which they are based. If we understand gender in this way, then it can be linked to violence both in the way that unequal gender structures underlie and cause violence and in so far as violence against women creates and reinforces gender inequalities. Thus, talking about the links between gender and violence requires 'attention to multiple aspects of gender and how these levels interact' (Anderson, 2009, p. 1452). To make this move towards an understanding of SGBV, which links all forms of violence against women to underlying structural socio-economic and political inequalities, it is vital to adopt a political economy approach (True, 2012). Rather than replacing the previously discussed research in public health, psychology, or criminology, such an approach can bring the missing links to fully understand and take action on SGBV. As True (2012) argues, political and economic inequalities shape women's vulnerability to violence in all settings. She thus advocates investigating the interconnectedness between the economic, social, and political realms to reveal the material bases of the use of violence (True, 2012).

## The Continuum of Violence

It is also important to understand and analyse the manifestations of SGBV along a continuum. The idea of a continuum of violence was first developed by Liz Kelly (1987) to describe the ways in which various forms of SGBV that women experienced across their lifetime were all different manifestations of the same phenomenon. As Kelly explains, during her research, 'it became clear that most women had experienced sexual violence in their lives. It was also clear that there was a range of possible experiences within each form of sexual violence discussed' (Kelly, 1987, p. 47). She thus understood a continuum as both 'a common character that underlies many different events' and 'a continuous series of elements or events that pass into one another and cannot be readily distinguished' (Kelly, 1987, p. 76). The existence of this continuum and the continual presence of various forms of violence in women's lives may also be seen to lead to a process of normalisation, whereby some of the supposedly more "minor" forms of SGBV, such as catcalls and sexist remarks, become part of everyday life for women and are no longer registered as violent. In our various studies, we can see how the continuums of violence play out in different ways. As with Kelly's initial study, we use the concept of the continuum to explain the ways in which SGBV manifests in various linked forms, including daily micro-aggressions, sexual harassment, sexual assault, rape, and many others.

All of these varying forms of violence are linked to underlying structures of inequality, are thus related and interlinked, and cannot be considered separately or as individual incidents. We also understand continuum as the ways in which violence plays out across women's lives, so that experiencing SGBV in childhood and young age is linked to continuing (and compounding) experiences of SGBV across the life course. Finally, we examine geographical continuums of violence, whereby SGBV is experienced as a continuum across geographical boundaries and borders (as is very clearly the case for women refugees, as we discuss below). These various continuums of violence play out in intersectional spaces and locations within different contexts.

As argued above, SGBV should not be understood as a series of isolated events or individual experiences but rather as a continuum of different forms and manifestations of violence, all rooted in structures of inequality. And as we have argued throughout this book, we need to adopt an intersectional lens to understand how and why women are placed in situations of particular vulnerability to this violence. Complex intersecting structures of inequality and domination create situations of vulnerability to violence but also entrap individuals in violence through limiting possibilities or increasing potential costs of disclosure (Rehman et al., 2016), restricting women's access to services and support, and also their opportunities for collective action. In the rest of the chapter, we trace these structurings of SGBV through research focusing on the experiences of various women who find themselves caught in these dangerous intersections. We begin with an analysis of the continuum of violence faced by women refugees in South Africa.

## Violence in and of Migration

One of the intersectional inequalities that emerged strongly from our research was that of having/not having legal status or citizenship in a country of residence. Turner refers to the importance of considering the "hierarchies of mobility" and the ways that women are frequently confined to the bottom rungs of this hierarchy, thus exposing them to a "dangerous intersection" (Turner, 2016, p. 60). This "dangerous intersection" was clearly visible in our research with women refugees in South Africa, which showed the various ways in which lack of legal status contributed to creating vulnerabilities for SGBV. As Krause (2017) argues, there is a dearth of research that investigates the continuum of violence for refugee women and that links the experiences of SGBV of refugees before, during, and after migration. In her article, she shows the impacts of this continuum across conflict, conflict-induced migration, and encampment in Africa. Our research in South Africa adds to this evidence by studying a continuum that links conflict, refugee migration, and settlement in a destination country with an urban refugee policy. Drawing on both feminist analyses of SGBV in conflict and on recent research of SGBV against women refugees during forced migration and in countries of destination (Freedman, 2016; Freedman et al., 2020), we explored how different forms of violence intersect and occur in a continuum, predisposing refugee women to interlocking cycles of violence in different settings of their migration experiences. We examine how structural inequalities that are inherent to the refugee experience in South Africa, such as the inability to obtain legal status, lack of accommodation, economic insecurities, and experiences of xenophobia and racism, exacerbate vulnerabilities to SGBV. We also seek to explore how the violence that women face at the different stages of refugee migration may make it more likely that they will experience varying forms of violence in their destination country.

Many women involved in our research had fled from situations of armed conflict, and their experiences of violence during these conflicts confirm existing research pointing to how there is a complex causal relationship between gendered inequality and discrimination, political violence, and SGBV (Davies & True, 2015). These women had often suffered from rape and other forms of violence in their countries of origin, which underpinned their decision to flee. SGBV experiences during conflict and post-conflict situations in their countries of origin were thus a key factor in influencing the women's decision to migrate and to seek refugee protection in another country. The conflict setting nature of this violence meant that women often departed their homes precipitously, with few economic resources to support them on their journey and with highly disrupted social and familial resources (Mutambara et al., 2023). Many women were travelling alone or accompanied only by their children because many of their husbands or families had been killed in conflict. This meant that women were located in situations where they were even more vulnerable to various forms of violence during their journeys and in transit to South Africa. While the prevalence of conflict disrupts social systems and pushes refugees to flee, those fleeing encounter hardships and challenges that continue to render them vulnerable to SGBV (Krause, 2017). Our research revealed that women refugees are exposed to different forms of violence on the long travel to their countries of destination and where sexual violence may be perpetuated by fellow refugees with whom they are travelling, from those facilitating the travel (e.g., truck drivers), or from border guards who demanded sex in exchange for entry into South Africa (Mutambara et al., 2023). One of the key informants from one of the organisations that support migrants and refugees told us that some of the women they had assisted reported to have used illegal channels and ports of entry, using the services of smugglers known as "malaisha" or "maguma guma" who were also frequently perpetrators of SGBV against the refugee women.

Many women did not obtain direct transport to South Africa and had to move from one place to the other through different country settings. This meant that some women refugees had to seek shelter in public spaces, like bus stops or on the streets, that were not safe and exposed them to opportunistic perpetration of sexual violence.

For women who are pregnant when they migrate or who become pregnant en route are faced with a lack of access to antenatal routine care and emergency care which can put their lives at risk. One woman we met who was pregnant at the time that she was forced to flee her country told us how she had no option but to give birth in the bushes with no medical care whilst on the run. Other women we interviewed were pregnant when they arrived in South Africa as a result of rape experienced in their country of origin or on their migration journey. In some cases, they did not even know that they were pregnant and found out by accident. One of these women asked a nurse based in South Africa to assist her with terminating the pregnancy because she did not want to keep the child in the circumstances. The nurse reportedly refused to give her any information on termination of pregnancy (TOP) services, even though TOPs are legally available on request in the country. The same woman also found out that she was now living with HIV. For women such as this, in addition to the trauma they experience as a result of the rape they have suffered, the fact of finding out that they are pregnant is an additional burden. The barriers to obtaining medical care, including access to safe abortion care when they request it, create another layer of stress and trauma for them.

On arriving in South Africa, refuge was not to be found for many women, as one Burundian woman explained: 'When I ran away from home, there was no safety and when I came to South Africa there is no safety; it's also happening here'. A combination of legal and economic insecurities, interacting with structures of gender inequality and xenophobia, results in a continuing state of insecurity and vulnerability for these women. We found that even "second generation" refugees who were born in South Africa or arrived at a very early age experienced vulnerabilities based on the intersection of legal, economic, and gendered inequalities (Crankshaw et al., 2023a).

The South African refugee policy allows asylum seekers to settle where they wish in the country while they attempt to make an asylum claim, rather than being restricted to a refugee camp or centre. However, despite the freedom that this offers it also means that they are left to fend for themselves with no State provision or support for accommodation, no economic support, or help with integration into the labour market, nor any psychosocial support to help them with any trauma they may have experienced or integration into South African society. This leaves many asylum seekers not only often highly traumatised but also extremely poor, often homeless, and lacking the means to provide for themselves, particularly if they have no pre-existing contacts or family in South Africa. Economic insecurities affect both men and women refugees, but our research found that women had more difficulty finding jobs in the informal labour market than men (Mutambara et al., 2023) and were thus more economically vulnerable.

Legal and economic insecurities led several of the women to stay with men who had either helped them to come to South Africa or who had approached them "to assist" while they were in precarious situations on arrival to the country (eg being abandoned in a strange city at night or found sleeping on the street). These situations created dependency and made them extremely vulnerable to violence. Even married or otherwise partnered women faced situations of violence where several women revealed that they had been victims of domestic violence, which some explained by their partners' anger about their constrained economic situations, and that the women were not earning any income. Previous research has shown increased levels of domestic violence against refugee and migrant women in their countries of destination (Menjívar & Salcido, 2002), which has been explained by changing gender relations during migration and also the stresses placed upon intimate partner relationships by the reception conditions in destination countries.

Key informants spoke about the fact that many of the refugee women they assisted were victims of domestic violence but that in most cases, women could not leave their relationships because of legal and economic dependencies. The research also found that those arriving in the country with their family are registered under one file holder at government Home Affairs offices, and in most cases, the file is registered in the name of the husband. This meant that for refugee women living in abusive relationships, leaving their partners would mean losing their refugee file status and jeopardising their chances of remaining documented (Mutambara et al., 2023).

Most of the women we interviewed were undocumented. In cases where women had been able to obtain asylum, they were given permits that only lasted 3–6 months, after which they would need to be renewed. Renewing asylum permits often required the need to travel long distances to the government office concerned but women also reported challenges in obtaining an appointment to do so. In cases where a husband had either left the family home or who had passed away, wives were unable to renew their claim since it is common practice for the man to be designated as the primary file holder. In their spouse's absence, women and their children had to start the refugee claim process all over again or were rendered undocumented and vulnerable.

Lack of legal documentation has huge impacts on women's lives and makes it difficult for them to obtain basic social services or employment, to get health care or to register their children in schools. This legal insecurity thus reinforced their vulnerabilities to violence and created obstacles to their accessing services if they were victims of violence.

The vulnerabilities of refugee women were deepened by their inability to pay for accommodation which led to homelessness and dependence on others. Several of the women we spoke to had difficulties finding and affording accommodation. Some of the women revealed that they were sleeping on the streets, and they were aware that this put them in an extremely vulnerable situation. One of the women recounted how she was almost raped because she had no shelter. Some of the women refugees who did not have accommodation got assistance from local shelters but sometimes these, in turn, exposed the women to risk and vulnerability for crime and SGBV. Shelters are also temporary solutions, some of which will only accommodate women for a maximum period of three months. These situations often created dependency on men or country mates who were willing to help. However, this also exposed women to sexual violence. In a focus group discussion with Congolese women, one woman had stopped speaking because of the traumatic incidents she had encountered. The other women who were staying with her explained that she fled the war, and when she arrived in Durban, she did not have a place to stay. She was assisted by a male pastor from one of the Congolese churches in Durban. However, she was raped by the pastor and had become pregnant as a result of the rape.

Violence was often also present in relationships and marriages which occurred after arrival in South Africa, with some male intimate partners using previous violent experiences to create forms of control and repeat victimisation. One of the women who had been raped by rebel soldiers in the DRC shared that when she and her male intimate partner argued, her partner would remind and shame her over her experience of rape. This was a constant source of hurt, and the woman felt that this past experience kept the window open for more abuse. Lack of economic resources, accommodation, or legal status also creates situations where women feel that marriage is one of their only choices, even at a very young age. In other cases, economic insecurity and a lack of livelihood options often leave women with little choice but to engage in sexual-economic exchange in order to survive. As with our other research, we found that this sexual-economic exchange had become the norm for women refugees. As discussed earlier in Chapter 3, none of the refugee women we interviewed identified as a sex worker or being involved in sex work. However, the above intersectional inequalities not only create vulnerabilities to violence but also an inability to leave or escape violent situations.

The experiences of refugee women clearly demonstrate both continuums of violence across geographical and temporal spaces and also the intersecting axes of inequality which create vulnerabilities to violence. In the following section, we explore other facets of these intersections and the ways in which they create vulnerabilities for SGBV across a continuum.

## Normalisation of Violence

Refugee women's experience is characterised by violence produced at the intersections of gender, a lack of legal status, economic insecurities, and xenophobia. But even for women with legal residence and citizenship status, the complex intersections of inequality lead to lifelong experiences of violence. In our various research projects, what was common across all countries and research contexts was the pervasiveness and continued experience of violence in women's lives. As evoked by the idea of a continuum of violence across their lifespan, these trajectories of violence took different forms but were rarely, if ever, once-off experiences. In many cases, violence is not even recognised as such, as it is understood as part of "normal" social behaviour and structures based on gendered roles and inequalities. This normalisation means that many women do not recognise it or name it as such. Even when they do name the violence that they have experienced, there remain barriers to reporting and to being taken seriously. The violence they experience is frequently minimised, and women have little to no recourse to justice. In what follows, we explore the manifestations of violence in various settings and the way that this is normalised and not reported as such in many cases, even by the women who experience it. Having experienced violence from an early age, many women just assume that this will be a part of their life experience.

### *Early Experiences of Violence*

Our research across the different countries underscored the continuum of different forms of violence and the ways in which they are deeply connected. We also noted a continuum of violence across women's lives, with violence beginning at a very early age and being normalised as part of women's experience (and man's perpetration of) as a result of this. In our research exploring the dynamics of SGBV amongst young women enrolled in tertiary education in the South African context, one female university student told us: 'I know four rape victims, who are people whom I'm close with or I was close with … the one person she was raped by an uncle … when she was eight this person decided to take advantage of her … then the other friend, she was, I think, she was four or seven years old when she was raped and it was also by a family member …'.

In Madagascar, we found that girls experienced SGBV from a very early age and that certain forms of violence were normalised as part of family relations. One young woman reported on a practice whereby fathers were expected to be the first men to have sex with their daughters.

> There are also those practices that have always existed, that it's a father who should "deflower" his daughter. Often, as the daughter grows up, she starts to wear clothes that show her body, and the father says, why should it be another man who is going to "open the champagne". That's a tradition, and there are still a lot of fathers that continue to do that. I know a girl who experienced that and she is still living with her father now.
>
> *(20-year-old woman, Madagascar)*

It was reported that in cases of intra-familial sexual violence, even when this was recognised as such, it was rarely reported for fear of bringing family into disrepute. Respondents explained that girls and women were discouraged from revealing any violence that they had experienced for fear of bringing shame on the family. One key informant working with adolescent girls in Zimbabwe echoed this situation:

> Communities have normalised (violence). It is (dealt with as) a private matter. Even when an adolescent has been raped by her father or uncle, we have cases where the mother encourages the daughter to keep quiet.
>
> *(Key informant, Zimbabwe)*

An estimated one-fifth of girls aged 15–19 have experienced forced sex during their lifetime (UNICEF, 2020). If sexual initiation occurs at a younger age, it is more likely to be forced (UNICEF, 2014). There are also links between child sexual abuse and unintended pregnancies. As mentioned in Chapter 3, in our research amongst young women who sell sex in Zambia, sexual debut was on average around 15 years of age but was reported to be as early as 11 years of age. And for at least one-tenth of our participants, sexual debut occurred in the form of sexual-economic exchange. Some young women shared that their sexual debut occurred as a result of sexual abuse. Child sexual abuse is highly gendered, with girls 2–3 times more likely to report sexual abuse than boys and with approximately 90% of perpetrators being male (UNICEF, 2020).

The students in our South African study provided insight into the fact that SGBV is normalised from a very young age, indicating also that it was widespread within the schools they attended as children. Young women talked about "boys travelling together" in a pack, reinforcing the acceptance of norms of dominant and aggressive behaviour against girls. They reflected on their experiences of feeling humiliated and degraded by groups of schoolboys catcalling and insulting themselves and/or other girls. This meant that girls learned to keep quiet and accept the behaviour. If they did complain, they were told that they were "overreacting". Male students in the same study confirmed these behaviours, with one male student sharing, 'We grew up seeing our uncles doing it and we are now doing it, I also think the next generation will also do it because it is our nature'. Indeed, undergraduate women students in our South African research expressed feelings of despair and anger over their everyday experiences of sexual harassment[3] in all aspects of their lives, underscoring the fundamental role of these "gender microaggressions" in the behavioural scaffolding of a "continuum of conduct" (Mothibi et al., 2013, p. 7) which may escalate into "high severity" forms of violence (physical and/or sexual). While sexual harassment is often invisible or underreported, it is always harmful because it is never a gender-neutral process; it is also a challenge that women overwhelmingly face (Benson & Thomson 1982). Indeed, definitions of the problem of sexual harassment as the 'widespread confluence of authority relations, sexual interest and gender stratification' (Benson & Thomson 1982, p. 238) cast categorisations of sexual harassment as "low severity" in a less benign light. Gartner and Sterzing (2016) further argue that gender microaggressions, which are deliberate or unintentional derogatory behaviours or speech based on gender, are environmental antecedents to, and overlap with, sexual harassment and assault. The normalisation and acceptability of such "micro-aggressions" create the context within which more "severe" forms of SGBV become frequent and, in turn, normalised. In patriarchal and gender unequal societies in all our research contexts, these gender microaggressions are the norm and should be viewed as part of the SGBV continuum.

We should thus understand a continuum of violence as not only encompassing widely diverse forms of SGBV but also stretching as a continuum across women's lifetimes. In all of our studies, our research showed the ways in which experiences of SGBV frequently started in early childhood and adolescence and then continued as women became young adults. Again, the vulnerabilities to all these different forms of SGBV as well as the availability of support or recourse to justice in the event of experiencing violence were structured by intersectional inequalities.

### *Synergistic Relationship between Sexual Economic Exchanges and SGBV*

Women are placed in situations of vulnerability to violence in function of their position in society within the intersectional web of inequalities. Our research across the region demonstrated the importance of economic status and income as a cause of vulnerability to SGBV. Lower socio-economic status and geographical marginalisation, interacting with unequal gender norms, were thus frequently linked to experiences of SGBV and poor SRHR. In Madagascar, our research showed that in poor and rural communities, lack of money combines with gender inequalities and traditional norms and leads families to encourage or push their daughters to have sexual relationships or to get married at an early age in order to be able to help support the family financially. As one respondent explained:

> There are also those cases where the girl is engaged to a young man as soon as she is born, practices that are still in force among some communities in the country. At around the age of 12–13, the young man's parents tell her parents that they are going to invite her to visit their village. So she goes and they put them together for the night while she is still a little girl who knows

nothing about what is going to happen to her. For me, this is also a form of violence!

*(18-year-old woman, Madagascar)*

This interviewee spoke about early marriages as a form of violence, but for others, the word was not used, and it was spoken about as a "normal" part of life.

In Zimbabwe, a push factor into selling sex was the absence of parents for those with orphanhood status. During the first wave of the HIV epidemic, mortality amongst adults was exceptionally high, with scores of young children surviving their parents, who either went on to manage a child-headed household or who found shelter with grandmothers or relatives. These household compositions were frequently described amongst our study participants who, in the context of deepening poverty, either lived with grandmothers who were now at an advanced age and often infirm with no source of income or who had lived with the relatives who had previously taken them in but could no longer afford to support them. These situations had directly led participants to engage in sexual-economic exchanges in order to survive. Other participants were heads of households that consisted of younger siblings who were entirely dependent on the household income that young women brought in through sexual-economic exchange. These trajectories are supported by the available evidence. According to the Zimbabwe National Statistics Agency, in 2018, about 13% of children <18 years old were orphans (Zimbabwe National Statistics Agency, 2018). The proportion of double orphans (where both biological parents are deceased) increases with orphan age, reaching a peak of 40.8% of the total number of double orphans in the 14–17 age group – the same age group as our study participants reporting entry into selling sex. Further, an earlier study amongst 836 adolescent girls (15–19 years) in Harare reported that half of their participants were single or double orphans and that experience of forced sex was high amongst all of the orphanhood groups (Birdthistle et al., 2008). In a later study, the same authors reported a link between childhood sexual abuse and subsequent entry into sex work (Birdthistle et al., 2011), highlighting the intersectional nature for vulnerability of orphaned adolescent girls.

Importantly, the same economic and social conditions that pushed young women into sexual economic exchanges in the first place created the very structures of violence in which SRHR vulnerabilities within this group occurred. For example, a precarious economic context, combined with gender inequalities, means that unprotected sex in exchange for higher payment is the norm rather than the exception. On the other end of the spectrum, non-payment for services – a rights-based challenge and a form of violence – was often accompanied by physical or sexual violence and theft, which further created vulnerability for poor SRH outcomes. Gender, age, and economic power differentials between young women and their male, often older, clients intersected in particular ways, which negatively impacted the negotiation around condom use and their ability to protect themselves from harm.

Young age, in particular, heightens vulnerability to violence and sexual exploitation, as was reflected on by a 20-year-old participant who was also engaged in selling sex:

> Younger sex workers do not have power, they submit to anything. If they are assaulted they go home and come back to work the next day.
>
> *(20-year-old woman, Zimbabwe)*

Young women expressed high awareness of the risks associated with unprotected sex, but these were overwhelmingly subordinate to economic concerns. The challenge of not being paid for services was raised frequently throughout the different focus group discussions in both Harare and Bulawayo[4] and evoked very strong response amongst participants. Sex without payment was often presented by them as being far worse than forced, unprotected sex, *with* payment. Experiences of violence, unprotected sex and non-payment often intersected with one another, over which young women were able to exercise little control. Young men, in particular, were mentioned as the main perpetrators of physical and sexual violence, as well as soldiers and illegal gold miners. In our Mozambique research, taxi drivers were also frequently mentioned as perpetrators, taking advantage of the late hours that the young women were travelling home and on their own.

Common across our research during COVID-19 in Zimbabwe and Mozambique were the impacts of the intersections of socioeconomic position and geospatial location on exposure to the experience of SGBV. An example of this were young women who sell sex of lower socioeconomic status/class who relied predominantly on being visible to clients by occupying physical space to meet clients. They reported greater experience of police harassment compared to the concealed, and therefore more secure, activities of adult sex workers who worked from home or in luxury hotels and used online platforms to contact clients (Aantjes et al., 2022). The closure of bars and heavy police surveillance also pushed these female sex workers into new areas of the city, where they operated in isolation and without protection against violent clients and street crime.

Our research in Zimbabwe carried out during the time of COVID-19 lockdowns cautions against reductionist understandings of vulnerability amongst marginalised populations, offering insight into the multifaceted inequalities amongst young people and how vulnerability played out both within and between young people of diverse genders and sexualities who were involved in sexual economic exchange (Crankshaw et al., 2023b). Our data highlighted the role of geographical spaces and gendered norms in creating and deepening vulnerabilities for some and not others. For example, among young people with diverse sexual orientation and gender identity, those with feminine identities were worst affected. In Zimbabwe, we found that those living in high-density, impoverished areas were the most negatively impacted by movement restrictions, with these areas being particularly heavily policed during the first lockdown and with reports of police violence and harassment (Crankshaw et al., 2023b). While all our research participants living in these areas were broadly impacted, cisgender and transgender women in particular were sexually harassed and sexually exploited, with transgender women reporting experiences of severe physical violence and sexual violence from law enforcement officials and clients. Important to our analysis is that our data also suggest that these experiences of violence were not unique to the lockdown period but part of a continuum of gender-based violence that existed in their daily lives well before the pandemic onset. These findings raise important questions about the obligations of a responsive state in reducing vulnerability and increasing resilience (Fineman, 2010) and in questioning the state's role in increasing vulnerability. The vulnerabilities associated with orphanhood raise similar questions.

## Recourse to Justice

As the above examples show, SGBV is widespread and experienced as a continuum across women's lives and in different forms. However, because of the normalisation of violence, there is, as we have argued, often a non-recognition that violence has occurred and also a reluctance to report violence. And if women do report violence, then frequently they are not able to gain any kind of recourse or justice. In many cases, SGBV may be dealt with "informally" through "amiable" resolutions and primarily through families with a focus on reconciliation (Medie, 2019). Medie (2019, p. 8) traces the presence of violence against women from colonial Africa to present-day Africa and notes that when violence is disclosed, 'it has mostly been to community and religious leaders. Although attitudes differ according to types of violence, the state has been called on and has intervened in only a minority of cases in most countries'.

In Madagascar, respondents talked about the ways that families would often "resolve" incidences of SGBV through negotiations with the perpetrator, sometimes involving him paying some form of compensation (often rice, cattle, and goats). In some cases, the victim of SGBV might also be pushed to marry the perpetrator in addition to this compensation. Local chiefs could also be called upon to resolve cases of SGBV, and here again, they were likely to try and find an "amiable" solution to preserve "good neighbourhood relations" (Freedman et al., 2021). This means that expectations of and recourse to justice will be lacking for many women who experience SGBV.

In many countries, there are reports of police not taking claims of SGBV seriously and doing nothing to prosecute perpetrators. This lack of police attention is clearly not just an African issue, but we did find that it was common across all of our country's research sites. In Madagascar, young women talked about the fact that the police would not take claims of SGBV seriously and would often blame the woman herself. In one case of a young woman who had been raped, for example:

> When she went to the police, she was still wearing the same clothes that she had been wearing when she was raped. The police asked the perpetrator what he had done, and he replied that the way that the young woman was dressed would arouse men. The police analysed her way of dressing and decided that her claim for rape would not stand up. The man was released immediately.
>
> *(Participant ID missing)*

Similar scenarios were reported in Zimbabwe, in the words of a 21-year-old young woman:

> Police do not take our cases seriously. They accuse us of looking for trouble by dressing provocatively or going to the bars. If you report a rape case they will ask you to put on the clothes you were wearing when you got raped. We wear short, revealing clothes when we go to work. So they will blame us. At the end it is useless to go to the police. It is a waste of time.
>
> *(21-year-old woman, Zimbabwe)*

Other young women in the Madagascar study evoked the fear of going to the police because they believed that the police themselves would be likely to commit acts of SGBV against them if they went to report it (Freedman et al., 2021). This situation also emerged in our Zimbabwean research, as the following 23-year-old participant shares: 'Women do not have power. Where can I report that I have been beaten up? Police officers will tell you that sex work violence does not involve them. Sometimes some officers will tell you that if you want your case to be attended then you have to sleep with them first'. Similarly, among women of diverse SOGIE, almost all said they would not consider taking legal action and were also advised not to do so by friends. They did not believe that police and judicial institutions would apply the laws to protect them and that if they were identified as having a diverse sexual orientation or gender identity, this could in fact lead to further violence from the police.

## Consequences of Violence

In the above sections, we have drawn attention to a number of manifestations of violence, particularly sexual and physical violence. However, we here also draw attention to the less tangible and therefore difficult-to-identify violence of emotional abuse. Key informants from civil society organisations in Zimbabwe spoke about the impact of the high levels of emotional violence that young women had to endure and the depression and cases of suicide that occurred as a consequence. A 20-year-old participant in Zimbabwe told us, 'I know I am a sex worker but sometimes clients treat us inhumanely, they take away our dignity. For example, you can get a client who can force you to have sex with them anywhere, in front of people, in the bushes, in the car, in the bar, anywhere. For me it is inappropriate. It takes away my dignity as a human being'. When asked whether she can say no to clients such as these, she replies: 'Saying no depends on two things. You are either prepared to get a beating or be ready to flee the scene. If you decide to run you should make sure that you will be changing your location because if you do not they will come back to seek their revenge'. In the same study, one key informant who provided psychosocial support to sex workers shared the weight of hearing the experiences of violence amongst these young women: 'When I was working in [name of informal settlement in Zimbabwe] we interacted with a lot of young sex workers … The first few days I would actually cry because I was not emotionally ready for it. I would cry. Some of them have a lot of stories that they have hidden and as sex workers you might think that they are ok. They seem strong but they are carrying pain, deep down there is a lot of pain'.

With a lack of recourse to justice, many young women will not share or report their experiences of violence, and our research found that this situation had a profound impact on women's self-esteem and self-worth. A number of young women in our Zimbabwe research shared having suicidal thoughts, with one young woman explaining why she had contemplated suicide: 'There are situations where I have lost hope!'. A key informant working on SGBV sensitisation and support in a sex worker organisation in Zimbabwe explained to us the way in which violence reinforced and deepened the already marginalised young women's standing in society in a way that could cause them to feel hopeless:

> If one lives in an abusive environment it negatively impacts their health. I also think that it impacts areas to do with personal development. If, for example, a young sex worker is being abused in whatever setting, there aren't laws protecting them, their dreams for a better future are silenced. They cannot even dream about being a better person or developing some skills. So it makes it very hard to have any form of personal development in their lives. They remain stagnant and they only dream of continuing in the profession, living like this. It has become their norm. But it is only because sometimes we might not see the physical harm but it is also internal. Some of them if you ask them to draw or write about what one sees beyond this life, they do not have a vision because of their experiences they have given up. That makes it

very hard for them to develop personally and even take part in other activities in the community. They can decide to sideline themselves which means that when it comes to decision-making tables, they will never be seen there. They always remain at the lowest position in the community because they look down on themselves.

Violence also leads to very poor SRH outcomes. The evidence suggests that repeated exposure to violence not only serves to normalise the violence but can also negatively impact decision-making around negotiating condom use with sexual partners (Shamu et al., 2019). Our and other research has highlighted the complex interactions between early and unintended pregnancy, IPV, HIV, and sexual-economic exchanges in the context of economic and social insecurities. A recent analysis of demographic health survey datasets in five countries in Africa reported that the association between experience of physical violence amongst pregnant adolescents was five-folds significant compared to non-pregnant adolescents (Tetteh et al., 2020). Physical violence was also highly associated with adolescent pregnancy in both directions, with early pregnancy occurring over four times more amongst adolescents who had ever experienced any form of physical violence compared to their peers who had never experienced physical violence (Ibid). The serious negative impacts of physical violence during pregnancy on maternal and infant health outcomes have been well established (Bailey, 2010; Chisholm et al., 2017; Murray et al., 2020). Experiences of childhood violence have been linked to an increased risk of HIV and other STIs and mental health problems, including substance use, depression, and stress (Lindert et al., 2014; Norman et al., 2012).

## Conclusion: Building Responses to Violence

In the previous sections, we have detailed the ways in which SGBV is pervasive and founded in intersecting structures of inequality. We can note that despite multiple international, regional, and national treaties, conventions, and laws, high levels of SGBV persist. So why is it seemingly so hard to tackle SGBV, and what else could be done? As Mannell et al. (2019, p. 4) argue, too many SGBV interventions are 'focused on tackling "risk factors" whether at the individual or structural level, rather than supporting women's agency, (which) can pose a major barrier for supporting changes in behaviour among young women because they often fail to recognize how gender and age inequalities intersect'. This idea of countering "risk" is, as we have argued throughout the book, limiting, as it individualises and medicalises SGBV and responses to it. The same holds true for gender-transformative interventions that target men to change their relationships or households as isolated cases (Dworkin & Barker, 2019). Instead, as we have argued in this chapter, we need to understand SGBV as produced by structural inequalities which must be changed. So how could SGBV be better addressed? To attempt to offer some answers, we return to our vulnerability analysis and to the understanding of vulnerability to violence as produced intersectionally and contextually, based on structures of economic, social, legal, and political gendered inequality. Analysing how women are rendered vulnerable to SGBV also opens up space for developing analysis for how they might become more resilient. This is not about promoting individual empowerment or resilience along the neo-liberal model but about how to change structural inequalities to ensure that resources for resilience are more equitably shared between women and men across different social classes, locations, sexual orientations, gender identities, etc. This also means that women should not be seen as "victims" but as agents who can mobilise against SGBV if they are provided with the space and resources to do so (Breton, 2022). In her work on vulnerability and resilience, Fineman stresses the role of the state in ensuring the redistribution of resources for resilience, and we argue that this redistribution is necessary to change the structures of inequality underlying vulnerability to SGBV and to provide women with just this space and these resources to be able to change the situation.

By improving the asylum system in South Africa, for example, to allow women fleeing SGBV to access refugee protection and legal status, the South African state would thus enable these women to access a variety of resources linked to this legal status and to mobilise their agency for resilience against SGBV. Similarly, redistributive economic policies, which help to reduce gendered economic inequalities, would help to provide the resources for all women to resist SGBV.

The state also has a role in helping to counter unequal gender norms, and one way this could be achieved would be through education programmes which work with children and young people to understand gender and sexuality and work towards more equal norms and representations. Education at an early age is also critical in primary sexual violence prevention, as some research suggests that many men who perpetrate sexual violence will do so for the first time in their teenage years (Heilman et al., 2014). It is therefore important to intervene early and reach girls and boys when their attitudes and beliefs about gender stereotypes and sexuality are still developing (Clare et al., 2021 Peacock & Barker, 2014). While schools have been found to be effective platforms for SGBV prevention intervention (Keith et al., 2023), few comprehensive sexuality education programmes have consistently addressed the concept of gender equality or approached gender and power in any depth. Globally as well as in sub-Saharan Africa, there is a growing body of evidence showing that gender norms can be transformed through curriculum-based programmes (Haberland & Rogow, 2015). Studies have demonstrated that adopting an approach that explicitly addresses issues of gender and power can have positive effects on learner sexual behaviours and sexual and reproductive health (SRH) outcomes (Haberland, 2015; Rogow & Haberland, 2005). Programmes that included a focus on transforming gender relationships and integrating discussions on gender power have been shown to be more effective than those programmes that do not include this focus. In a 2015 review of evaluated studies, a focus on transforming gender and power was found to be a key characteristic of effective sexuality and HIV education programmes, with the programmes that addressed gender or power being five times more likely to be effective and 80% of these programmes associated with lower rates of STIs or unintended pregnancies (Haberland, 2015). Ten of the total 22 reviewed interventions were school-based, out of which two reduced pregnancy rates; these two were the only ones that addressed gender or power in the school subgroup (Haberland, 2015). The review also highlighted that to transform gender norms, information alone is not sufficient (Rogow & Haberland, 2005). Interactive, learner-centred, and skills-based pedagogies are also key characteristics linked to effective programmes (Kirby, 2007). In the above review, the effective interventions shared common ground in the way that they explicitly addressed gender and power and facilitated critical thinking around these topics. They also employed participatory and learner-centred pedagogies and encouraged critical reflection over how gender and power play out in the personal and social domains (Haberland, 2015). Developing critical thinking skills amongst learners enables boys and girls to meaningfully engage with the ways that gender shapes their lives and sexual relationships (Rogow & Haberland, 2005). Critical reflection of the socialisation of gender roles has the potential to change sexual attitudes and subsequent behaviours (Rogow & Haberland, 2005).

These are just some of the ways that states and governments can work with women to combat SGBV by tackling underlying structures of inequality and providing spaces for women to mobilise and use collective agency and resilience against violence. SGBV interventions must work with women, listening to them and understanding the resources that they need to combat the structures which render them vulnerable.

## Notes

1 Africa has its own set of regional conventions and policies which have been praised as a strong response to the high prevalence of SGBV on the continent. The Protocol to the African Charter on Human and Peoples' Rights, on the Rights of Women in Africa, also known as the Maputo Protocol, prohibits gender-based violence as part of women's rights to life, integrity and security of the person, and dignity. SADC has also put into place a regional level framework for tackling SGBV, with a Regional Strategy and Framework of Action (2018–2030) for addressing Gender-Based Violence.

2 https://www.ohchr.org/en/instruments-mechanisms/instruments/declaration-elimination-violence-against-women.

3 Sexual harassment includes sexual hostility, unwanted sexual attention, and sexual coercion.

4 Harare is the capital and most populous city in north-eastern Zimbabwe in the country's Mashonaland region. Bulawayo is the second largest city in the western part of Zimbabwe and the largest city in the country's Matabeleland region.

## References

Aantjes, C., Muchanga, V., & Munguambe, K. (2022). Exposed and unprotected: Sex worker vulnerabilities during the COVID-19 health emergency in Mozambique. *Global Public Health*, *17*(12), 3568–3582.

Anderson, K. L. (2009). Gendering coercive control. *Violence Against Women*, *15*(12), 1444–1457.

Bailey, B. A. (2010). Partner violence during pregnancy: Prevalence, effects, screening, and management. *International Journal of Women's Health*, 2, 183–197.

Benson, D. J., & Thomson, G. E. (1982). Sexual harassment on a university campus: The confluence of authority relations, sexual interest and gender stratification. *Social Problems*, *29*(3), 236–251. https://doi.org/10.2307/800157

Birdthistle, I. J., Floyd, S., Machingura, A., Mudziwapasi, N., Gregson, S., & Glynn, J. R. (2008). From affected to infected? Orphanhood and HIV risk among female adolescents in urban Zimbabwe. *AIDS*, *22*(6), 759–766.

Birdthistle, I. J., Floyd, S., Mwanasa, S., Nyagadza, A., Gwiza, E., & Glynn, J. R. (2011). Child sexual abuse and links to HIV and orphanhood in urban Zimbabwe. *Journal of Epidemiology and Community Health*, *65*(12), 1075–82.

Breton, N. N. (2022). Reflecting on our good intentions: A critical discourse analysis of women's health and empowerment discourses in sexual and gender-based violence policies relevant to southern Africa. *Global Public Health*, 18(1), 1–16.

Chisholm, C. A., Bullock, L., & Ferguson, J. E. J. II (2017). Intimate partner violence and pregnancy: Epidemiology and impact. *American Journal of Obstetrics and Gynecology*, *217*(2), 141–144.

Clare, C. A., Velasquez, G., Martorell, G. M. M., Fernandez, D., Dinh, J., & Montague, A. (2021). Risk factors for male perpetration of intimate partner violence: A review. *Aggression and Violent Behavior*, *56*, 101532.

Cornwall, Harrison, & Whitehead (2007). Cornwall, A., Harrison, E., & Whitehead, A. (2007). Gender myths and feminist fables: The struggle for interpretive power in gender and development. *Development and Change*, *38*(1), 1–20.

Crankshaw, T. L., Freedman, J., & Mutambara, V. M. (2023a). Intergenerational trajectories of inherited vulnerabilities amongst young women refugees in South Africa. *Comparative Migration Studies*, *11*(1), 1–18.

Crankshaw, T. L., Muparamoto, N., Chareka, S., & Ngwenya, P. (2023b). Intersectional vulnerabilities and differential impacts of COVID-19 responses on young people who sell sex in Zimbabwe. *Culture, Health & Sexuality*, *25*(7), 818–832.

Davies, S. E., & True, J. (2015). Reframing conflict-related sexual and gender-based violence: Bringing gender analysis back in. *Security Dialogue*, *46*(6), 495–512.

Dworkin, S. L., & Barker, G. (2019). Gender-transformative approaches to engaging men in reducing gender-based violence: A response to Brush & Miller's "Trouble in Paradigm. *Violence Against Women*, *25*(14), 1657–1671.

Fineman, M. A. (2010). The vulnerable subject and the responsive state. *EmoRy lJ*, *60*, 251.

Freedman, J. (2016). Sexual and gender-based violence against refugee women: A hidden aspect of the refugee" crisis. *Reproductive Health Matters*, *24*(47), 18–26.

Freedman, J., Crankshaw, T. L., & Mutambara, V. M. (2020). Sexual and reproductive health of asylum seeking and refugee women in South Africa: Understanding the determinants of vulnerability. *Sexual and Reproductive Health Matters*, *28*(1), 1758440.

Freedman, J., Rakotoarindrasata, M., & de Dieu Randrianasolorivo, J. (2021). Analysing the economies of transactional sex amongst young people: Case study of Madagascar. *World Development*, *138*, 105289.

Garcia-Moreno, C. (2002). Dilemmas and opportunities for an appropriate health-service response to violence against women. *The Lancet*, *359*(9316), 1509–1514.

Gartner, R. E., & Sterzing, P. R. (2016). Gender microaggressions as a gateway to sexual harassment and sexual assault: Expanding the conceptualization of youth sexual violence. *Affilia*, *31*(4), 491–503.

Graaff, K. (2021). The implications of a narrow understanding of gender-based violence. *Feminist Encounters*, *5*(1), 1–12.

Greig, A. (2011). Chapter seventeen anxious States and directions for masculinities work with men. *Men and Development*, *219*.

Haberland, N. A. (2015). The case for addressing gender and power in sexuality and HIV education: A comprehensive review of evaluation studies. *International Perspectives on Sexual and Reproductive Health*, *41*(1), 31–42.

Haberland, N., & Rogow, D. (2015). Sexuality education: Emerging trends in evidence and practice. *Journal of Adolescent Health*, *56*(1), S15–S21.

Hayes, C. (2007). Tackling violence against women: A worldwide approach. *Gender-Based Violence*, 1

Heilman, B., Hebert, L., & Paul-Gera, N. (2014). The making of sexual violence: How does a boy grow up to commit rape? Evidence from five IMAGES countries. International Center for Research on Women (ICRW). https://www.icrw.org/wp-content/uploads/2016/10/The-Making-Of-Sexual-Violence-June-2014-WEB-PREVIEW.pdf

Hughes, C., Marrs, C., & Sweetman, C. (2016). Introduction to gender, development and VAWG. *Gender & Development*, *24*(2), 157–169.

Inter-Agency Standing Committee. (2015). Guidelines for Integrating Gender-based Violence Interventions in Humanitarian Action: Reducing risk, promoting resilience and aiding recovery. Available at: https://gbvguidelines.org/wp/wp-content/uploads/2015/09/2015-IASC-Gender-based-Violence-Guidelines_lo-res.pdf

Jakobsen, H. (2014). What's gendered about gender-based violence?: An empirically grounded theoretical exploration from Tanzania. *Gender and Society*, *28*(4), 537–561. http://www.jstor.org/stable/43669907

Jewkes, R. (2002). Intimate partner violence: Causes and prevention. *The Lancet*, *359*(9315), 1423–1429.

Keith, T., Hyslop, F., & Richmond, R. (2023). A systematic review of interventions to reduce gender-based violence among women and girls in sub-Saharan Africa. *Trauma, Violence, & Abuse*, *24*(3), 1443–1464.

Kelly, L. (1987). "The continuum of sexual violence. In J. Hanmer, & M. Maynard (Eds.), *Women, violence and social control. Explorations in sociology* (British Sociological Association Conference Volume series). Palgrave Macmillan.

Kirby D. (2007). Emerging answers: Research findings on programs to reduce teen pregnancy and sexually transmitted diseases. National Campaign to Prevent Teen and Unplanned Pregnancy.

Krause, U. (2017). Escaping conflicts and being safe? Post-conflict refugee camps and the continuum of violence. *Gender, Violence, Refugees*, *173*.

Leach, F., & Humphreys, S. (2007). Gender violence in schools: Taking the 'girls-as-victims' discourse forward. *Gender & Development*, *15*(1), 51–65.

Lindert, J., von Ehrenstein, O. S., Grashow, R., Gal, G., Braehler, E., & Weisskopf, M. G. (2014). Sexual and physical abuse in childhood is associated with depression and anxiety over the life course: Systematic review and meta-analysis. *International Journal of Public Health*, *59*(2), 359–72.

Mannell, J., Willan, S., Shahmanesh, M., Seeley, J., Sherr, L., & Gibbs, A. (2019). Why interventions to prevent intimate partner violence and HIV have failed young women in southern Africa. *Journal of Internation AIDS Soc*, *22*(8), e25380. doi: 10.1002/jia2.25380. PMID: 31441229; PMCID: PMC6706780.

Medie, P. A. (2019). Women and violence in Africa. In *Oxford Research Encyclopedia of African History*. Oxford University Press.

Menjívar, C., & Salcido, O. (2002). Immigrant women and domestic violence: Common experiences in different countries. *Gender & Society*, *16*(6), 898–920.

Mothibi, J., Naicker, V., Meyersfeld, B. and Omar, J. (2013). Independent inquiry into allegations of sexual harassment at the University of the Witwatersrand, Johannesburg. https://www.wits.ac.za/media/wits-university/faculties-and-schools/commerce-law-and-management/research-entities/cals/documents/programmes/gender/Final%20Report%20Independent%20Inquiry%20into%20Sexual%20Harassment%20at%20Wits%20University%203%20September%202013.pdf

Murray, A. L., Kaiser, D., Valdebenito, S., Hughes, C., Baban, A., Fernando, A. D., Madrid, B., Ward, C. L., Osafo, J., Dunne, M., Sikander, S., Walker, S., Van Thang, V., Tomlinson, M., & Eisner, M. (2020). The intergenerational effects of intimate partner violence in pregnancy: Mediating pathways and implications for prevention. *Trauma Violence Abuse*, *21*(5), 964–976. doi: 10.1177/1524838018813563. Epub 2018 Dec 4. PMID: 30514180.

Mutambara, V. M., Freedman, J., Crankshaw, T. L., & Rajah, Y. (2023). Gendered insecurities: Exploring the continuum of sexual and gender-based violence experiences of refugee women in South Africa. In: Freedman, J., Latouche, A., Miranda, A., Sahraoui, N., Santana de Andrade, G., Tyszler, E. *The gender of borders* (pp. 103–118). Routledge.

Norman, R. E., Byambaa, M., De, R., Butchart, A., Scott, J., & Vos, T. (2012). The long-term health consequences of child physical abuse, emotional abuse, and neglect: A systematic review and meta-analysis. *PLOS Medicine*, *9*(11), e1001349.

Peacock, D., & Barker, G. (2014). Working with men and boys to prevent gender-based violence: Principles, lessons learned, and ways forward. *Men and Masculinities*, *17*(5), 578–599.

Ratele, K. (2014). Hegemonic African masculinities and men's heterosexual lives: Some uses for homophobia. *African Studies Review*, *57*(2), 115–130.

Read-Hamilton, S. (2014). Gender-based violence: A confused and contested term. *Humanitarian Exchange Magazine*, *60*(February), 5–8.

Rehman, Y., Kelly, L., & Siddiqui, H. (2016). *Moving in the shadows: Violence in the lives of minority women and children*. Routledge.

Rogow, D., & Haberland, N. (2005). Sexuality and relationships education: Toward a social studies approach. *Sex Education*, *5*(4), 333–344.

Scully, P. (2009). Vulnerable women: A critical reflection on human rights discourse and sexual violence. *Emory International Law Review*, *23*, 113.

Scully, P. (2010). Expanding the concept of gender-based violence in peacebuilding and development. *Journal of Peacebuilding & Development*, *5*(3), 21–33.

Shamu, S., Shamu, P., Zarowsky, C., Temmerman, M., Shefer, T., & Abrahams, N. (2019). Does a history of sexual and physical childhood abuse contribute to HIV infection risk in adulthood? A study among post-natal women in Harare, Zimbabwe. *PLOS One*, *14*(1), e0198866.

Shefer, T., Stevens, G., & Clowes, L. (2010). Men in Africa: Masculinities, materiality and meaning. *Journal of Psychology in Africa*, *20*(4), 511–517.

Terry, G. (2007). *Gender-based violence*. Oxfam GB.

Tetteh, J., Nuertey, B. D., Dwomoh, D., Udofia, E. A., Mohammed, S., Adjei-Mensah, E., & Yawson, A. E. (2020). Teenage pregnancy and experience of physical violence among women aged 15-19 years in five African countries: Analysis of complex survey data. *PloS One*, *15*(10), e0241348.

True, J. (2012). *The political economy of violence against women*. Oxford University Press.

Turner, C. (2016). *Violence, law and the impossibility of transitional justice*. Routledge.

UNICEF (2014). *Hidden in plain sight: A statistical analysis of violence against children*. United Nations Children's Fund.

UNICEF. (2020). *Action to end child sexual abuse and exploitation*. UNICEF.

World Health Organisaiton. (2021). *Violence against women prevalence estimates, 2018: Global, regional and national prevalence estimates for intimate partner violence against women and global and regional prevalence estimates for non-partner sexual violence against women*. World Health Organisation.

World Bank (2023). *Unlocking the potential of women and adolescent girls challenges and opportunities for greater empowerment of women and adolescent girls in Madagascar*. World Bank.

Zimbabwe National Statistics Agency. (2018). Poverty, Income, Consumption and Expenditure Survey 2017 Report. http://www.zimstat.co.zw/sites/default/files/img/publications/National%20Accounts/PICES_2017%20Final_Report_2019.pdf

# 6 CONCLUSION

## Introduction

Our book has argued that a continuing focus on HIV and a medicalised and "risk" reduction approach has led to an ongoing neglect of wider sexual and reproductive health and rights (SRHR) issues. This means that women, and especially young women within the Southern African region, continue to find themselves vulnerable to various negative SRH outcomes. We have described the ways in which colonial discourses around the dangers and "risks" of the spread of infectious diseases, which stigmatised African sexualities and in particular women's sexual behaviour, have morphed into Eurocentric bio-medical discourse, which prolongs this notion of HIV as a major "risk" which needs to be contained. To do so, a treatment approach has been developed, focusing on those "most at risk" or "key populations". This approach, we have argued, has reduced the scope of SRHR policies and programmes, failing to fully take into account the ways in which HIV and AIDS are embedded in and linked to the whole range of SRHR. And whilst it is true that Southern Africa is one of the regions of the world which is most affected by HIV and AIDS, the continuing focus on HIV has drawn attention and funding away from other issues, which we have argued are in fact more crucial to ensuring good SRHR (including better HIV outcomes) for the majority of women in the region. The call to better understand the various matrices of inequalities that create vulnerability may be unappealing for some, where there is a real temptation to invest in treatment at the expense of prevention. However, the intractable problem of new HIV infections in the region provides a clear indication that treatment alone is not sufficient. The SRHR agenda calls for a holistic approach in which HIV is one part

DOI: 10.4324/9781003414698-6

of a number of other linked and pressing health concerns, and to address these, we need to understand how the various inequalities operate.

We argue that the individualised "risk" reduction approach leads to solutions proposing that individuals take responsibility for their own "resilience", a neoliberal approach which neglects the structural and systemic causes of vulnerability. Rather than understand vulnerability in terms of "vulnerable groups" or "key populations", we have proposed an understanding based on the idea that everyone is potentially vulnerable and that actual vulnerability is caused by a system of intersecting inequalities. Individuals find themselves located in vulnerable situations within this dynamic matrix of inequality. And to escape or resist this vulnerability, they cannot rely on individual "resilience" but need state-led intervention to provide resources and reduce the inequalities and domination which they face. For example, our study of refugee women showed how a lack of access to asylum protection and the failure to provide any material support frequently lead to women engaging in sexual-economic exchange both to gain legal status, shelter, and economic support. This clearly makes them vulnerable to negative SRHR outcomes. A fully functioning asylum and refugee policy – and one which treats women's cases as independent and not as part of their male partner's asylum application – would help to reduce vulnerabilities for these women.

In parallel to providing resources, states can work towards decriminalising punitive colonial-era laws which police behaviours and which often impede the realisation of rights and access to health services where young people and women are disproportionately negatively impacted (for example, through age of consent laws and access to safe abortion care – both of which directly constrain women's reproductive choices).

Our research pointed to the salience of some factors of inequality, particularly economic inequalities. We explored in Chapter 3, for example, the ways in which economic inequality intersects with gender norms to constrain women's choices around sexual-economic exchanges and how a continuum of forms of sexual-economic exchange are rooted in economic inequalities. And in Chapter 5, we also showed how economic inequality is linked to vulnerability to sexual and gender-based violence (SGBV) and to a lack of resources (and resilience) to be able to escape situations of violence. Economic inequalities intersect with persistent forms of gender inequality and domination. Strong gender norms persist around women's sexual behaviour and fertility, which may lead to family pressures to become pregnant or marry at an early age, as discussed in Chapter 4. The intersections of sex and gender in increasing vulnerability play out in very specific ways for women of reproductive age, and particularly young women, and the vulnerabilities created by these intersections of sex and gender are not experienced by men. Pregnancy and, ultimately, being financially responsible for child dependents, often in the absence of the fathers, was common across study settings. These gendered inequalities in norms around childbearing and childcare force many women into situations of deep economic insecurity, which in turn reinforces their intersectional vulnerability to poor SRH. The fact that the region faces the parallel challenge of high rates of early and unintended pregnancies and high adolescent birth rates together with ongoing HIV infections provides clear evidence of the deepening intersections of vulnerability for young girls and women and makes a strong case to bring HIV back into the constellation of SRHR, where vulnerability is understood as complex and not just as individual risk behaviour.

Another important finding from our research was the importance of age as a social category of inequality. Many intersectional approaches tend to neglect age as a social category or instead talk about generation as a category of analysis (Crankshaw et al., 2023), but our findings point to the ways in which young age is a significant factor in vulnerability in a number of ways. Young women engaged in sexual-economic transactions, for example, were found to be exploited and discriminated against by older women as well as by men. And these young women were often unable or unwilling to access services dedicated to sex workers, even when they self-identified as such, because these services were dominated by older women. Similarly, young women's difficulties in accessing contraceptive services without first having borne a child highlight an intersection between gender inequalities, age, and concomitant access to care.

Legal systems also create structures of inequality, as our example of refugee women shows. Not having legal residence status or citizenship status is an important factor in creating situations of vulnerability for women and may push them into sexual-economic exchanges, create vulnerabilities to SGBV and other poor SRH outcomes, and lead to them staying in violent relationships as they are made dependent on men for both legal and economic status. And legal systems which criminalise sex work and/or abortion effectively criminalise women themselves by creating vulnerabilities for those women who need to terminate their pregnancies for a variety of reasons, as well as limiting access to termination by creating fear amongst health professionals. It is well known that women living in sub-Saharan Africa are the most likely to die from complications arising from unsafe abortions compared to women living in any other world region (Bankole et al., 2019). And it is no coincidence that those countries with the most restrictive abortion laws also have the highest rates of maternal mortality and higher adolescent birth rates.

If we understand vulnerability as a result of situated intersectional inequalities, then it is clear that the response to this is complex. Rather than proposing an overarching solution such as "HIV treatment" targeted at a few pre-defined groups based on a set of assumptions, we argue that improving SRHR involves a deep and located understanding of the intersecting factors of vulnerability in different local contexts. This means leaving behind the idea that there are groups who are essentially "at risk" or "a risk" and moving towards an understanding that the most vulnerable and marginalised are those who find themselves at the centre of a matrice of inequalities and that this matrice will vary over time and geographical location. It is then impossible to talk about "vulnerable groups" per se. Instead, vulnerability is understood to be situated in time and space. Having carried out research and inquiry to understand how intersecting vulnerabilities act to marginalise certain people, it is then possible to develop policies to reduce vulnerability and improve resilience by increasing the amounts of resources available to those in the most vulnerable situations. These resources are not just economic but also social and relational. Meaning that the interlinked economic and legal inequalities and gender and age inequalities all need to be addressed. It is not enough merely to invest money in a programme without understanding the social structures and norms within which the programme will operate and the ways in which these also increase inequalities. To return to the example of young women who self-identified as involved in selling sex, it is not enough to create programmes for "sex workers" and invest money in them without understanding the ways that gender norms and age interact with economic inequalities to render young women particularly vulnerable in this case. These young women may not even access the programmes for reasons that we have detailed previously in the book.

A first step towards ensuring better SRHR for young women is thus to complexify our understandings and to stop trying to seek simplistic categorisations of those "at risk", but rather to understand the ways in which individuals become more or less vulnerable across their lifetime as a result of intersecting inequalities. This understanding could guide where interventions would best be targeted to reach those most marginalised and vulnerable.

Having made this argument about the complexities of vulnerability, we feel that it is important to conclude the volume by discussing a major issue for current and future societies which will act to reinforce and deepen inequalities even further, that of climate change. In the following sections, we will discuss the current state of knowledge on how climate change impacts the SRHR of women in the Southern African region and tie the central themes reflected in this volume, such as SGBV and migration, into our discussion.

## Gendered Vulnerabilities to Climate Change

The previous chapters of this book have discussed the various ways in which women are placed in positions of vulnerability to poor SRHR due to intersecting structures and systems of domination and inequality. A major issue which must be considered in assessing vulnerabilities now and in the future is the impact of climate change. Given its enormous impact on health, Chersich et al. (2018) suggest that climate change could and should be reframed as predominantly a health issue. Global research has already shown the differential vulnerabilities caused by climate change in terms of health outcomes, with women and girls in particular experiencing greater vulnerability (Women Deliver, 2021). Climate change has already begun to deepen existing inequalities, and in doing so, it will contribute to the matrix of intersecting inequalities, creating vulnerabilities for poor SRHR. As van Daalen et al. (2021, p. 1) argue, 'Worldwide, women and girls face increased climate-induced health risks compared to men and boys. This is mainly a result from greater exposure and susceptibility to natural hazards and climate-related damage as well as less ability to respond to health impacts, due to cultural and societal norms, including in dimensions of sexual and reproductive health'. And research is beginning to emerge linking climate change to various important impacts on SRHR, including SGBV, increasing rates of sexual-economic exchange, and limiting access to HIV care. As Women Deliver found in a report linking climate change and SRHR, 'Significant evidence points to how climate change, and particularly climate-related disasters, can be linked to increased vulnerability to GBV, including sexual violence, transactional sex, and sex trafficking. In turn, these are linked to increased risk of sexually transmitted infections and unintended pregnancies' (Women Deliver 2021, p. 7).

## The Impacts of Climate Change in the Southern African Region

The Intergovernmental Panel on Climate Change has called Africa 'one of the most vulnerable continents to climate variability and change because of multiple stresses and low adaptive capacity' (IPCC, 2007, p. 10). This finding was echoed in the African Union Climate Change and Resilient Development Strategy and Action Plan (2022–2032), which states that Africa is 'one of the regions that are most vulnerable to climate variability and change. This is due to the continent's biophysical makeup as well as numerous socio-economic vulnerabilities – including a high dependence on rain-fed agriculture (and natural resource-based sectors broadly), a lack of alternative livelihood support, widespread poverty and inequality, weak adaptive capacity, low levels of education, and inequitable access to financial resources, credit, markets, and climate information services (CIS)' (African Union, 2023, p. 3). Climate change is expected to increase the likelihood of both sudden-onset events such as major flooding and more long-term disasters such as drought, sea-level rise, and coastal erosion (Zickgraf, 2019). And within the continent, Southern Africa is a region which has been identified as being particularly impacted by climate change because of its geographical location. The impacts of climate change are also amplified by the existing levels of poverty and inequality in the region. It is an already warm and dry region, and warming in the interior of

Southern Africa is occurring at about twice the global average rate (Scholes & Engelbrecht, 2021). This entails high risks for agricultural production, both in the reduction of the production of staple crops such as maize and of livestock (Scholes & Engelbrecht, 2021). And as Thoithi et al. (2021) suggest, the highly variable rainfall across Southern Africa disproportionately affects the poor rural population that is heavily dependent on rain-fed agriculture for food production.

Climate change has been widely linked to migration, with a variety of climate impacts leading people to migrate either nationally (from rural to urban areas) or internationally across borders. There is a lack of accurate statistics and data to quantify this migration (Zickgraf, 2019), and indeed, migration often has a variety of causes, of which climate change is only one. However, research suggests that climate change is playing an increasing role as a driver of migration (Jilesen & Wegerif, 2023), and it is highly likely that climate change will continue to increase migration within the Southern African region, both in the form of displacement following rapid-onset disasters and more gradual migration linked to drought, low agricultural yields, and increasing poverty and inequality resulting from these. And although climate migration is a reality, little is known about the specific SRHR needs and challenges linked to climate migration. As van Daalen et al. (2021, p. 2) argue, 'This is a particular concern due to the potential "risk-multiplier" effect of compounding vulnerabilities of climate change and migration, and a challenge due to the lack of research and operation consensus in defining climate migration'.

We have shown, for example, in previous chapters the specific vulnerabilities faced by women migrants, particularly in terms of increased exposure to SGBV and the likelihood of engaging in sexual-economic exchanges. Increasing migration linked to climate-induced poverty and inequality will only serve to increase the numbers of women on the move and place them in added situations of vulnerability. Further, those "left behind" will also face increasing vulnerabilities. Research has shown, for example, that in Northern Mozambique, where drought has collided with ongoing conflict, women were less able to engage in mobility due to fears of conflict-related sexual violence and thus remained trapped in poverty and unable to adapt or respond to their situation (Lubkemann, 2008; Zickgraf, 2019). A study in Zambia on the impacts of drought also showed gendered patterns of migration, with men more likely to migrate out of drought-affected areas, leaving women behind to look after the children. These female-headed households were found to be left in extremely vulnerable positions (Rosen et al., 2021). And similar outcomes were shown by research in Madagascar, which showed that men migrated out of the drought-affected area of Androy to seek work in other areas of the country. This left women as heads of household and in a particularly vulnerable position supporting a household of dependants (Randriamparany & Randrianalijaona, 2022). The research shows that traditional structures and norms of gender inequality, such as early marriage, contribute to women's vulnerability but are also reinforced by drought, so that women become even more vulnerable.

Climate change is also linked to conflicts, which can in turn lead to migration and displacement. The interaction between the environment and conflict is complex and diverse, 'taking the form of disagreements at local level ... that these can become outright wars and even lead to genocide' (Jaggernath, 2014, p. 91). Jaggernath (2014) also shows the gendered nature of climate-related conflict in Africa, arguing that environmentally induced conflicts undermine women's asset base, leading to increased vulnerability to displacement, conflict-induced migration, and SGBV. Further, climate change-induced mobility/migration is not only a response to conflicts and tensions in one location, but it also promotes conflicts in receiving locations as a result of competition over resources, ethnic tensions, and distrust (Reuveny, 2007).

## Sexual Economies and Climate Change

In Chapter 3, we discussed the issue of sexual-economic exchange as an important SRHR issue in the region. An emerging body of research is showing the links between climate change and the economies of sexual exchange (Fiorella et al., 2019). This builds on existing research describing the links between the availability of natural resources (such as fish) and sexual-economic exchange (Béné, & Merten, 2008). In communities reliant on natural resources, gender inequalities generally make women most vulnerable to the scarcity of these resources, and there is already literature describing the ways in which these scarcities lead to sexual-economic exchange as a means of economic survival for women and their families (Fiorella et al., 2019).

Treibich et al. (2022) draw a direct link between drought and an increase in sexual-economic exchange in Malawi. They show that women working in agriculture are highly sensitive to the impacts of drought on their income and that drought conditions push a real increase in the proportion of women engaging in sexual-economic exchanges. They also show that this leads to a significant increase in these women's vulnerability to sexually transmitted infections. Their results highlight 'the additional vulnerability faced by women relying on agriculture, in particular women who have low education and limited labour opportunities' (Treibich et al., 2022, p. 9). A recent modelling exercise testing the relationship between increased temperatures and HIV prevalence found that men report an increase in sexual partners and engagement in paid sex over a warmer period (Baker, 2020). This may be related to men's migration for work opportunities due to climate change (Baker, 2020).

Climate change leads to increasing food insecurity, and there is a significant body of evidence that shows that food insecurity can increase vulnerability to sexual-economic exchange, unprotected sex, early sexual debut and marriage, forced sex, and a number of sexual partners (Khalifa et al., 2022; Bellandi, 2022; Epstein et al., 2022; Low et al., 2022). Our research conducted during the COVID pandemic showed a relationship between food insecurity and increased vulnerability to poor SRH. In Zimbabwe, female sex workers told us that they felt they had "no choice" but to accept extremely low amounts in exchange for services (Crankshaw et al., 2023). The data suggested that the younger female participants were the most exposed to sexual exploitation and were unlikely to insist on protection against HIV and other STIs.

## Climate Change and SGBV

In Chapter 5, we discussed how pervasive SGBV is in the Southern African context and, more broadly, its impacts on SRHR. Women and girls are disproportionately negatively impacted by natural disasters in their experience of violence and exploitation (Thurston et al., 2021). In their systematic review of the links between natural disasters and violence against women and girls, Thurston and colleagues (2021) found that close to half of the quantitative studies reported an association with increased IPV across all income settings, suggesting a direct relationship between disaster exposure and the perpetuation of IPV. These findings suggest that we may expect deepening inequalities in settings with already existing poor SGBV indicators. Of note, their review found that no studies reported decreased levels of SGBV following a disaster exposure. Drawing on the qualitative study insights, the authors hypothesise three different pathways between disaster exposure and vulnerability to SGBV, which include heightened stressors that catalyse SGBV, an environment that enables SGBV, and an increase in the underlying drivers of SGBV. Economic insecurity emerged as a major catalyst for the perpetuation of SGBV and simultaneously deepened women's vulnerability to experience violence since they feared reporting or leaving their intimate partner on whom they were financially dependent (Ibid). Meyiwa et al. (2014), in their research with rural women in communities in the Eastern Cape and KwaZulu-Natal on climate change, found that young girls are exposed to gender-based violence because they are forced, as a result of climate change, to search further and further from home for water.

Climate change has also been linked to an increase in the prevalence of early marriage. A study in Zambia, for example, showed how drought led to increased levels of early marriages for girls as young as 12 as parents sought to reduce the number of dependents in the household (Rosen et al., 2021). One respondent in this research explained that 'People used to get married at the right age, like 25 years and above. But this time, children as young as 12 years-old are forced into early marriages in order for their parents to survive' (cited in Rosen et al., 2021, p. 8). Other studies have also found an increase in forced early marriage of girls following a climate disaster (Thurston et al., 2021).

## Climate Change and SRH Outcomes

Changes in environmental variables, such as temperature and rainfall, have a direct influence on human behaviours, disease pathogens, and vectors and may, consequently, alter the incidence, distribution, and spread of disease in a given area (De Souza et al., 2012). The early impacts of climate change on SRHR have led to rising concerns about the "climate crisis-HIV nexus" (Lieber et al., 2021; Williams et al., 2024) and the urgent need for increased HIV prevention interventions. Climate change has been linked to HIV transmission in Lesotho due to poverty resulting from food insecurity and impacts on livelihoods (Braun, 2020; Low et al., 2022). In Malawi, a study found that a single drought increased HIV prevalence around 15% (Treibich et al., 2022). A modelling exercise testing the effect of temperature changes on HIV prevalence found that warmer periods were linked with an increase in HIV prevalence, particularly amongst younger groups, and predicted between 11.6 and 16 million new cases of HIV by 2050 (Baker, 2020). An earlier modelling found that HIV infection rates in rural areas across countries in Sub-Saharan Africa increased by 11% for every recent drought (Burke et al., 2015).

This has led to a surge of interest in the provision of biomedical technologies, such as pre-exposure prophylaxis products, that are "climate resilient" in that they are driven by user preference, don't rely on health facility service delivery models, and are resistant to extreme weather (Williams et al., 2024). However, many of these approaches continue to risk marginalising the linked SRH challenges, such as the concomitant need for contraceptive methods to prevent unintended pregnancy or access to safe abortion care in situations where a pregnancy is unwanted. Family planning services have been shown to have been disrupted by climate change disasters. For example, Rosen et al. (2021) found that in Zambia, family planning services were particularly susceptible to drought-related disruption, resulting in high contraceptive discontinuation rates.

### Impacts on Access to SRH Services

It is well established that global economic inequalities impact people's ability to access SRH services (Bearak et al., 2020), and since climate change is set to worsen these economic inequalities, a resulting impact on access to SRH services is to be expected. Equally, health services will increasingly come under pressure with a greater burden of health challenges brought on by extreme weather events and water shortages, such as malnutrition, infectious disease outbreaks, non-communicable diseases, heat-related illnesses and deaths, and poor mental health (Lokotola et al., 2023; World Bank, 2023). Further, it is expected that populations will become increasingly mobile as they seek more hospitable living environments. This means that health systems are required to prepare and invest in climate-proofing of health facilities, the provision of innovative health service delivery for mobile populations, and the development of climate-resilient products and packaging for drugs (Williams et al., 2024; World Bank, 2023). It is also expected that there will be a decline in economic growth in developing countries (Adom, 2024). It is anticipated that before 2050 there will be moderate economic loss in the medium term, but that this will increase substantially with some country-level projections ranging from 11.2% to 26.6% of GDP in the long term in the most impacted regions of Africa (Adom, 2024). Most countries in sub-Saharan Africa do not currently have adequate domestic resources for health financing and fall well below the Abuja target set by the African Union in 2001. In the context of existing weak health systems and a lack of adequate financing for health, countries in the region may not have the ability to respond to and be agile in delivering the necessary services for climate-driven health challenges in the future.

Further, despite the evident need for continued investment in SRHR services, these may be neglected following climate disasters, when more "pressing" health concerns are prioritised. A UNFPA report (2021) argues that when disasters or emergency situations occur, health resources are diverted towards combating them and away from services that are considered less essential, including sexual and reproductive health. This was clearly visible during the COVID-19 pandemic, when women's health was impacted by deepening gender inequality and SRHR services were often neglected in favour of diverting resources to vaccine programmes (Marzouk et al., 2023). The COVID-19 response can be viewed as a precursor to understand how health systems will fare in the face of increasingly frequent climate emergencies, with already under-resourced health systems being hit the hardest. The de-prioritisation of SRHR services in these emergency situations can be seen as very short termist, as the neglect of SRHR services will have serious impacts, particularly on women's health and rights (Malakar et al., 2023).

## Concluding Remarks

The available research and evidence show the major negative impacts of climate change on women's SRHR in Southern Africa. With the world unlikely to meet agreed targets on climate change mitigation efforts, it can be anticipated that these negative SRHR impacts will only worsen in the coming years, adding to inequalities and vulnerabilities. In order to try and counter some of these negative effects and find strategies for improving women's SRHR despite climate change, it is imperative to include women in discussions and planning for how best to promote resilience. Wonders (2018), for example, argues that the connections between climate change and gender inequalities call for an integration of climate justice and gender justice. This includes improving inclusive decision-making processes, as gendered vulnerability is inextricably linked with access to resources. In including women in decision-making processes, however, essentialist forms of gender inclusion which position women as "closer to nature" must be avoided. As Resurrección (2013) notes, these types of discourses only act to shift the burden of environmental care onto women. Thinking about climate justice and gender justice should lead to a real integration of gender equality concerns into national adaptation plans for climate change (Burns & Mutunga, 2024), including a focus on SRHR as an essential component of gender equality and women's rights. Returning once again to the main argument of our book, climate change and the increasing frequency of climate-linked disasters add another layer of complexity, which will increase gender inequalities and thus deepen situations of vulnerability. It is vital to understand these complex pathways into vulnerability in order to better plan programmes and services which will address these vulnerabilities and support real resilience for those made most vulnerable.

## References


Adom, P. K. (2024). *The socioeconomic impact of climate change in developing countries in the next decades: A review*. CGD Working Paper 681. Center for Global Development. https://www.cgdev.org/publication/socioeconomic-impact-climate-change-developing-countries-next-decades-review

African Union. (2023). African Union climate change and resilient development strategy and action plan (2022-2032). https://au.int/sites/default/files/documents/41959-doc-CC_Strategy_and_Action_Plan_2022-2032_08_02_23_Single_Print_Ready.pdf

Baker, R. E. (2020). Climate change drives increase in modeled HIV prevalence. *Climatic Change*, *163*(1), 237–252.

Bankole, A., Remez, L., Owolabi, O., Philbin, J., & Williams, P. (2020). *From Unsafe to Safe Abortion in Sub-Saharan Africa: Slow but Steady Progress*. GuttmacherInstitute. https://www.guttmacher.org/report/from-unsafe-to-safe-abortion-in-subsaharan-africa

Bearak, J., Popinchalk, A., Ganatra, B., Moller, A. B., Tunçalp, Ö, Beavin, C., Kwok, L., & Alkema, L. (2020). Unintended pregnancy and abortion by income, region, and the legal status of abortion: Estimates from a comprehensive model for 1990–2019. *The Lancet Global Health*, *8*(9), e1152–e1161.

Bellandi, D. (2022). An association between heavy rainfall and HIV in Sub-Saharan Africa. *JAMA*, *328*(15), 1490. https://doi.org/10.1001/jama.2022.15476.

Béné, C., & Merten, S. (2008). Women and fish-for-sex: Transactional sex, HIV/AIDS and gender in African fisheries. *World Development*, *36*(5), 875–899.

Braun, Y.A. (2020). Environmental change, risk and vulnerability: poverty, food insecurity and HIV/AIDS amid infrastructural development and climate change in Southern Africa. *Cambridge Journal of Regions, Economy and Society*, *13*(2), 267–291. https://doi.org/10.1093/cjres/rsaa008

Burke, M., Gong, E., & Jones, K. (2015). Income shocks and HIV in Africa, *The Economic Journal*, *125*, 1157–1189, https://doi.org/10.1111/ecoj.12149

Burns, P. A., & Mutunga, C. (2024). Addressing the impact of climate change on sexual and reproductive health among adolescent girls and young women in low-and middle-income countries. *Global Health: Science and Practice*, *12*(1).

Chersich, M. F., Wright, C. Y., Venter, F., Rees, H., Scorgie, F., & Erasmus, B. (2018). Impacts of climate change on health and wellbeing in South Africa. *International Journal of Environmental Research and Public Health, 15*(9), 1884.

Crankshaw, T. L., Freedman, J., & Mutambara, V. M. (2023). Intergenerational trajectories of inherited vulnerabilities amongst young women refugees in South Africa. *Comparative Migration Studies, 11*(1), 10.

De Souza, D. K., Owusu, P. N., & Wilson, M. D. (2012). Impact of climate change on the geographic scope of diseases. In Chettri (Ed.), *Human and social dimensions of climate change*. Intech.

Epstein, A., Nagata, J. M., Ganson, K. T., Nash, D., Saberi, P., Tsai, A. C., Charlebois, E. D., & Weiser, S. D. (2022). Drought, HIV testing, and HIV transmission risk behaviors: A population-based study in 10 high HIV prevalence countries in Sub-Saharan Africa. *Aids and Behavior, 27*(3), 855–863. https://doi.org/10.1007/s10461-022-03820-4

Fiorella, K. J., Desai, P., Miller, J. D., Okeyo, N. O., & Young, S. L. (2019). A review of transactional sex for natural resources: Under-researched, overstated, or unique to fishing economies? *Global Public Health, 14*(12), 1803–1814.

IPCC. (2007). Climate change 2007: Synthesis report. Contribution of working groups I, II and III to the fourth assessment report of the intergovernmental panel on climate change [Core Writing Team, Pachauri, R.K and Reisinger, A. (eds.)].

Jaggernath, J. (2014). Women, climate change and environmentally-induced conflicts in Africa. *Agenda - Empowering Women for Gender Equity, 28*(3), 90–101.

Jilesen, R., & Wegerif, M. (2023). Climate, environment and migration: Experiences of migrants in South Africa. *Afrika Focus, 36*(2), 195–222.

Khalifa, A., Findley, S. E., Gummerson, E., Mantell, J. E., Hakim, A., Philip, N. M., Ginindza, C., Hassani, A. S., Hong, S. Y., Jalloh, M. F., Kirungi, W., Maile, L., Mgomella, G., Miller, L. A., Minchella, P., Mutenda, N., Njau, P., Schwitters, A., Ward, J., & Low, A. (2022). Associations between mobility, food insecurity, And transactional sex among women in cohabitating partnerships: An Analysis from 6 African countries 2016–2017. *Journal of Acquired Immune Deficiency Syndromes, 90*(4), 388–398. https://doi.org/10.1097/qai.0000000000002995

Lieber, M., Chin-Hong, P., Whittle, H. J., Hogg, R., & Weiser, S. D. (2021). The synergistic relationship between climate change and the HIV/AIDS epidemic: A conceptual framework. *AIDS and Behavior, 25*, 2266–2277.

Lokotola, C. L., Mash, R., Naidoo, K., Mubangizi, V., Mofolo, N., & Schwerdtle, P. N. (2023). Climate change and primary health care in Africa: A scoping review. *The Journal of Climate Change and Health, 11*, 100229.

Low, A., Gummerson, E., Schwitters, A., Bonifácio, R., Teferi, M., Mutenda, N., Ayton, S., Juma, J., Ahpoe, C., Ginindza, C., Patel, H., Biraro, S., Sachathep, K., Hakim, A., Barradas, D. T., Hassani, A. S., Kirungi, W., Jackson, K., Goeke, L., … & Findley, S. E. (2022). Food insecurity and the risk of HIV acquisition: Findings from population-based surveys in six sub-Saharan African countries (2016–2017). *BMJ Open, 12*(7), e058704. https://doi.org/10.1136/bmjopen-2021-058704

Lubkemann, S. C. (2008). Involuntary immobility: On a theoretical invisibility in forced migration studies. *Journal of Refugee Studies, 21*(4), 454–475. https://doi.org/10.1093/jrs/fen043

Malakar, K. D., Kumar, M., Anand, S., & Kuzur, G. (2023). Climate change, justice, and rights. In *Climate change and socio-ecological transformation: Vulnerability and sustainability* (pp. 375–437). Springer Nature Singapore.

Marzouk, M., Lam, S. T., Durrance-Bagale, A., Nagashima-Hayashi, M., Neo, P., Ung, M., Zaseela, A., Aribou, Z. M., Agarwal, S., & Howard, N. (2023). Effects of COVID-19 on sexual and reproductive health services access in the Asia-Pacific region: A qualitative study of expert and policymaker perspectives. *Sexual and Reproductive Health Matters*, 1, 2247237. https://doi.org/10.1080/26410397.2023.2247237.

Meyiwa, T., Maseti, T., Ngubane, S., Letsekha, T., & Rozani, C. (2014). Women in selected rural municipalities: Resilience and agency against vulnerabilities to climate change. *Agenda*, *28*(3), 102–114.

Randriamparany, S. T., & Randrianalijaona, T. M. (2022). The vulnerability of Antandroy women to droughts in Ambovombe Androy (Madagascar). *International Journal of Disaster Risk Reduction*, *72*, 102821.

Resurrección, B. P. (2013). Persistent women and environment linkages in climate change and sustainable development agendas. *Women's Studies International Forum*, *40*, 33–43. https://doi.org/10.1016/j.wsif.2013.03.011.

Reuveny, R. (2007). Climate change-induced migration and violent conflict. *Political Geography*, *26*, 656–673.

Rosen, J. G., Mulenga, D., Phiri, L., Okpara, N., Brander, C., Chelwa, N., & Mbizvo, M. T. (2021). "Burnt by the scorching sun": Climate-induced livelihood transformations, reproductive health, and fertility trajectories in drought-affected communities of Zambia. *BMC Public Health*, *21*(1), 1–14.

Scholes, R., & Engelbrecht, F. (2021). *Climate impacts in southern Africa during the 21st century. Report for earth justice and the centre for environmental rights*. Global Change Institute, University of Witwatersrand.

Thoithi, W., Blamey, R. C., & Reason, C. J. (2021). Dry spells, wet days, and their trends across Southern Africa during the summer rainy season. *Geophysical Research Letters*, *48*(5), e2020GL091041.

Thurston, A. M., Stöckl, H., & Ranganathan, M. (2021). Natural hazards, disasters and violence against women and girls: A global mixed-methods systematic review. *BMJ Global Health*, *6*(4), e004377.

Treibich, C., Bell, E., Lépine, A., & Blanc, É (2022). From a drought to HIV: An analysis of the effect of droughts on transactional sex and sexually transmitted infections in Malawi, *SSM-Population Health*, *19*, 101221, https://doi.org/10.1016/j.ssmph.2022.101221

van Daalen, K. R., Dada, S., Issa, R., Chowdhury, M., Jung, L., Singh, L., Stokes, D., Orcutt, M., & Singh, N. S. (2021). A scoping review to assess sexual and reproductive health outcomes, challenges and recommendations in the context of climate migration. *Frontiers Global Women's Health*, 2:757153. https://doi.org/10.3389/fgwh.2021.757153.

Williams, K. M., Olisa, A. L., & Wilcher, R. (2024). Exploring linkages: Addressing the relationship between the climate crisis and HIV prevention with recommendations for emerging pre-exposure prophylaxis programs. *Frontiers in Reproductive Health*, *6*, 1369762.

Women Deliver. (n.d). The Impact of COVID-19 on Sexual and Reproductive Health and Rights: Youth-led Perspectives and Solutions for a Gender-Equal World. http://womendeliver.org/wp-content/uploads/2022/05/FULL-REPORT.pdf

Women Deliver (2021). *The link between climate change and sexual and reproductive health and rights*. Women Deliver, Available at: https://womendeliver.org/wpcontent/uploads/2021/02/Climate-Change-Report-1.pdf.

Wonders, N. A. (2018). Climate change, the production of gendered insecurity and slow intimate partner violence. In *Intimate partner violence, risk and security* (pp. 34–51). Routledge.

World Bank. (2023). Health and Climate Change: Brief. Accessed 2 April 2023: https://www.worldbank.org/en/topic/health/brief/health-and-climate-change.

Zickgraf, C. (2019). *Climate change and migration crisis in Africa*, in C. Menjívar, M. Ruiz, and I. Ness (eds.; pp 347–364). The Oxford Handbook of Migration Crises. Oxford University Press.

# INDEX